The Menopause Journey

From Symptoms to Solutions

A short introduction by The HealthSpan Institute

The Menopause Journey:
From Symptoms to Solutions

ISBN: 9798867411312

Copyright © 2023 Wellness Press

Printed in the United States of America

Contents

Chapter 2:
The Science of Menopause

Chapter 3:
Common Symptoms and Their Causes

Chapter 4:
Medical Management of Menopause

Chapter 5:
Lifestyle Approaches to Managing Symptoms

Chapter 6:
Holistic and Alternative Therapies

Chapter 7:
Emotional Well-being and Mental Health

Chapter 8:
Navigating Relationships and Sexuality

Chapter 9:
Planning for a Healthy Future

Chapter 10:
Stories from the Journey

Chapter 11:
Resources and Tools for the Journey

Chapter 12:
Conclusion

Chapter 1: Introduction– Understanding the Menopause Journey

Overview of Menopause as a Natural Life Stage

Menopause marks a significant milestone in a woman's life, symbolizing the end of her reproductive years. It is not just a medical condition but a natural life stage every woman experiences. This chapter delves into understanding menopause as an integral part of a woman's journey, shedding light on its biological, emotional, and cultural aspects.

The Biological Perspective

Biologically, menopause is defined as the cessation of menstruation for twelve consecutive months, signaling the end of a woman's natural fertility. This transition typically occurs between the ages of 45 and 55, with the average age being around 51 years in most countries. However, the journey towards menopause, often termed as perimenopause, can begin several years earlier, characterized by irregular menstrual cycles, hormonal fluctuations, and various physical symptoms.

The primary biological change during menopause is the decline in the production of estrogen and progesterone, hormones produced by the ovaries. These hormones play a vital role in regulating menstruation and ovulation during the reproductive years. As a woman approaches menopause, the ovaries gradually reduce their hormone production, leading to various physiological changes.

Understanding Symptoms

The fluctuation and eventual decline in hormone levels can lead to a range of symptoms. The most common include hot flashes, night sweats, mood swings, sleep disturbances, and changes in libido. While these symptoms are widely acknowledged, their intensity and impact can vary significantly from one individual to another. Some women might experience mild discomfort, while others may face severe disruptions impacting their daily life.

It is important to recognize that menopause is a unique experience for each woman. Factors like genetics, lifestyle, overall health, and cultural attitudes can influence how one navigates through this phase. Hence, understanding menopause requires a personalized approach, acknowledging the diversity of experiences among women.

Emotional and Psychological Aspects

Menopause is not just a physical transition; it also encompasses emotional and psychological dimensions. For many women, entering menopause can elicit mixed emotions–relief from ending menstrual cycles and contraceptive concerns, or anxiety about aging and loss of fertility. This period can also bring about a sense of liberation or a time for self-reflection and personal growth.

The emotional response to menopause is often intertwined with societal attitudes and personal beliefs about aging and femininity. In some cultures, menopause is celebrated as a time of freedom and wisdom, while in others, it may be viewed with apprehension or stigma.

Menopause in the Modern Context

In today's society, where life expectancy has significantly increased, a woman may spend a considerable portion of her life in post-menopause. This shift has transformed menopause from being a brief phase to a substantial life stage, warranting greater attention and understanding.

The modern view of menopause is evolving. It is increasingly seen as a time for renewal and an opportunity to focus on self-care and health. With the right information and support, women can manage menopausal symptoms effectively and lead fulfilling lives.

The Role of Support and Education

Educating women about menopause and providing support are crucial. Knowledge about what to expect can alleviate fears and misconceptions. Healthcare providers play a pivotal role in offering accurate information and treatment options. Additionally, support from family, friends, and peer groups can significantly impact a woman's experience of menopause.

Support groups and forums have emerged as vital platforms for sharing experiences and advice. These communities not only offer emotional support but also empower women with knowledge and coping strategies.

Conclusion

Menopause, a natural life stage, marks a significant transition in a woman's life. It encompasses biological changes, emotional nuances, and cultural implications. By understanding menopause in its entirety, women can better prepare for and navigate this phase with confidence and positivity.

As we continue to explore the various facets of menopause in subsequent chapters, it's crucial to keep in mind that menopause is not an end but a new beginning. It's a stage where women can redefine themselves, focus on their health, and embrace the wisdom that comes with this phase of life. With a supportive environment and the right resources, the menopause journey can be a fulfilling and empowering experience.

Brief History and Cultural Perspectives on Menopause

Menopause, often referred to as the "change of life," is not merely a biological process but also a cultural and historical phenomenon. It has been experienced and interpreted in diverse ways across different cultures and historical periods. In this section, we explore the historical evolution of societal attitudes towards menopause and how various cultures perceive this significant life stage.

Historical Context

Historically, menopause has been both mystified and misunderstood. In ancient times, it was often not well-documented due to the shorter life expectancy of women and the limited understanding of female biology. However, as life expectancy increased and medical science advanced, menopause gained more attention.

In the 19th and early 20th centuries, menopause was often pathologized. It was viewed through a medical lens, primarily as a deficiency disease due to the reduction in estrogen production. This period saw menopause being associated with a variety of physical and mental ailments, often leading to stigmatization and misconceptions.

Menopause in Medical Literature

The first recorded mention of menopause dates back to Ancient Greece, where it was recognized but not thoroughly understood. In the 1700s, French physician de Gardanne coined the term "menopause" and it was during this time that menopause started to be seen as a distinct medical condition. However, the understanding of menopause was limited, often shrouded in myths and misconceptions.

The 20th century witnessed a significant shift in the medical community's approach to menopause. The development of hormone replacement therapy (HRT) in the 1960s was a pivotal moment, offering relief from menopausal symptoms and shifting the narrative towards managing menopause more effectively.

Cultural Perceptions and Variations

The cultural interpretation of menopause varies widely. In many Western societies, menopause has often been associated with aging and loss of femininity, contributing to negative attitudes. The societal emphasis on youth and beauty can make the transition to menopause particularly challenging for women in these cultures.

Conversely, in some Asian and African cultures, menopause is seen positively. For instance, in Japan, menopause (referred to as "konenki") is often viewed as a time of liberation and potential for personal growth. Similarly, in certain Indigenous cultures, post-menopausal women are revered as wise elders, playing crucial roles in community leadership and decision-making.

The Influence of Media and Society

Media portrayal has significantly influenced societal attitudes towards menopause. In much of the 20th century, menopause was often depicted in a negative light, with a focus on the loss of youth and fertility. However, in recent decades, there has been a gradual shift. Media and popular culture are beginning to portray menopause more positively, emphasizing empowerment, and celebrating this phase as a time of maturity and wisdom.

The Modern Perspective

In the modern era, there is a growing movement to destigmatize menopause and promote a more holistic understanding of it. This shift is driven by increasing awareness and open discussions about women's health. Women are more empowered to speak about their experiences, challenging outdated stereotypes and advocating for better healthcare and support.

Conclusion

The historical and cultural perspectives on menopause reveal a journey from misunderstanding and stigma to a growing appreciation and respect for this natural life stage. This evolution reflects broader changes in society's understanding of women's health and aging. As we continue to challenge stereotypes and promote open conversations, menopause can be redefined not as a time of loss but as a stage of renewal and empowerment.

Understanding these diverse perspectives is crucial in shaping how we approach menopause today. Recognizing menopause as a natural and significant phase in a woman's life allows for a more supportive, informed, and compassionate approach to this transition. As we move forward, it is essential to continue fostering a culture that values and respects the menopause journey, viewing it as an integral part of a woman's life experience.

The Importance of Open Conversations About Menopause

Menopause, a natural stage in a woman's life, has long been shrouded in silence and misunderstanding. It's a subject that, despite affecting half the population, often remains hidden in the shadows of societal taboos. The importance of open conversations about menopause cannot be overstated, as they are crucial for demystifying this life stage, promoting better health outcomes, and fostering a supportive and understanding society. This section explores why breaking the silence around menopause is vital for women's health and well-being.

Breaking the Taboo

Historically, menopause has been a taboo subject in many societies. This silence stems from a variety of cultural, social, and psychological factors, including misconceptions about aging, femininity, and sexuality. The reluctance to discuss menopause openly has led to a lack of awareness and understanding, leaving many women unprepared for its onset and unsure about how to manage its symptoms.

Open conversations about menopause serve to break this taboo. By talking openly about menopause, we can normalize it as a natural part of aging, just like puberty or pregnancy. This normalization is vital for changing societal attitudes and removing the stigma that many women face during this time.

Education and Awareness

Lack of knowledge about menopause can lead to fear, anxiety, and misconceptions. Many women enter menopause without knowing what to expect, which can make the experience more challenging. Open conversations facilitate better education and awareness, providing women with the information they need to understand the changes happening in their bodies.

Educational discussions can also extend to families, partners, and workplaces, fostering a more supportive environment for women going through menopause. By understanding menopause, others can empathize with and accommodate the needs of menopausal women, whether at home or in the workplace.

Health and Well-being

Menopause can bring a range of physical and psychological symptoms that vary in severity from woman to woman. Open conversations are crucial for women to recognize these symptoms as normal and seek appropriate medical advice and support. Discussing menopause openly can lead to better health outcomes, as women become more proactive in seeking treatment and making lifestyle adjustments to manage their symptoms effectively.

Moreover, discussing menopause can highlight related health concerns, such as increased risks of osteoporosis and heart disease, prompting women to take preventive health measures.

Empowerment and Solidarity

Open discussions about menopause can be incredibly empowering. They provide a platform for women to share their experiences, challenges, and successes, creating a sense of community and solidarity. This collective sharing can be a powerful tool in combating isolation and fostering a sense of belonging among women undergoing similar experiences.

Furthermore, open conversations can empower women to advocate for themselves in healthcare settings, ensuring they receive the care and attention they need. It can also drive demand for more research and better healthcare options for menopausal women.

Mental Health Considerations

Menopause can be a significant psychological transition for many women, often coinciding with other life changes such as children leaving home or caring for aging parents. Open conversations about the emotional and psychological aspects of menopause are crucial for mental health. Recognizing and addressing feelings of loss, anxiety, or depression associated with menopause can help women navigate this transition more smoothly.

Workplace Implications

As more women stay in the workforce longer, understanding menopause becomes increasingly relevant in the workplace. Open conversations can lead to better workplace policies and accommodations for menopausal women, such as flexible working hours or temperature control. This understanding can create a more inclusive and supportive work environment, enhancing productivity and job satisfaction.

Conclusion

The importance of open conversations about menopause extends far beyond individual experiences; it is about creating a society that acknowledges and supports women through all stages of life. By discussing menopause openly, we can foster a culture that respects and values the health and well-being of women, recognizes the diversity of their experiences, and supports them in navigating this significant life transition.

Encouraging open dialogues about menopause can transform it from a whispered-about issue into a shared journey of empowerment and understanding. As we progress through this book, we will explore the various facets of menopause, aiming to provide a comprehensive guide that not only educates but also empowers women to approach menopause with confidence and positivity.

Chapter 2: The Science of Menopause

Biological Changes During Menopause

Menopause is often perceived as merely the end of menstruation, but it's a profound biological shift that encompasses much more. This natural transition in a woman's life, typically occurring between the ages of 45 and 55, is marked by significant hormonal changes that can have wide-ranging effects on health and well-being. In this blog post, we'll explore these biological changes that occur during menopause, shedding light on their impacts and implications.

The Hormonal Roller Coaster

The hallmark of menopause is the fluctuation and eventual decline in key female hormones, primarily estrogen and progesterone. These hormones have played pivotal roles throughout a woman's reproductive life, regulating everything from the menstrual cycle to the health of various tissues in the body. As menopause approaches, the ovaries gradually reduce their production of these hormones, leading to several noticeable changes.

The decrease in estrogen levels is particularly significant. Estrogen is involved in numerous bodily functions, and its reduction can lead to various symptoms and long-term health implications. Progesterone levels also decline during this period, contributing to the cessation of menstruation and affecting the body in various ways.

Menstrual Irregularity and Cessation

One of the first signs of approaching menopause is a change in the menstrual cycle. Periods may become irregular, with variations in flow and duration before stopping altogether. This irregularity is due to the ovaries gradually producing less estrogen and progesterone, leading to anovulatory cycles (cycles where ovulation does not occur) and eventually, the end of menstrual periods.

Vasomotor Symptoms

Perhaps the most talked-about symptoms of menopause are hot flashes and night sweats, known as vasomotor symptoms. These sudden feelings of intense heat in the upper body, accompanied by sweating and sometimes a rapid heartbeat, can be uncomfortable and disruptive. They result from the body's thermostat (located in the hypothalamus) becoming more sensitive to slight changes in body temperature due to hormonal fluctuations.

Vaginal and Urinary Changes

Lower estrogen levels can lead to thinning and drying of the vaginal walls, a condition known as vaginal atrophy. This can cause discomfort during intercourse, an increased risk of vaginal infections, and sometimes urinary symptoms. The urinary tract also undergoes changes during menopause, which can lead to increased frequency of urination and a higher risk of urinary tract infections.

Long-term Health Considerations

Menopause has several long-term health implications, primarily due to the decreased production of estrogen. One of the most significant concerns is the increased risk of osteoporosis. Estrogen helps maintain bone density, and its reduction can lead to bones becoming weaker and more prone to fractures. This makes it essential for postmenopausal women to pay attention to their bone health, including adequate intake of calcium and vitamin D and engaging in weight-bearing exercises.

Another major concern is the increased risk of cardiovascular disease post-menopause. Estrogen has a protective effect on the heart and blood vessels, and its decline can lead to changes that increase the risk of developing heart-related conditions.

Managing the Changes

Understanding and managing the biological changes of menopause can significantly impact how women experience this transition. For some, hormone replacement therapy (HRT) can be a way to alleviate symptoms by replacing the hormones the body no longer makes. However, HRT is not suitable for everyone, and it's important to discuss its benefits and risks with a healthcare provider.

Lifestyle adjustments also play a crucial role in managing menopause symptoms and reducing long-term health risks. A balanced diet, regular exercise, and stress management techniques can help alleviate symptoms and improve overall health. Additionally, treatments like vaginal moisturizers and lubricants can help manage vaginal dryness, making sexual activity more comfortable.

The Psychological Aspect

The hormonal changes during menopause can also affect mental health, potentially leading to mood swings, anxiety, or depression. Seeking support when needed, whether from healthcare professionals, support groups, or counseling, is crucial.

Embracing the Transition

Menopause is more than just a biological process; it's a significant life transition. It's a time that can be filled with growth, self-discovery, and new opportunities. By understanding the biological changes that occur during menopause and adopting strategies to manage them, women can embrace this phase of life with confidence and positivity. This period can mark the beginning of an enriching, empowering chapter, offering a chance to focus on personal health, well-being, and happiness.

The Stages of Menopause: Perimenopause, Menopause, and Postmenopause

Menopause is not an event but a gradual process that unfolds in distinct stages, each with its own set of characteristics and challenges. Understanding these stages – perimenopause, menopause, and postmenopause – is vital for any woman approaching or experiencing this transition. This blog post aims to demystify these stages, providing insight into what to expect and how to navigate each phase effectively.

Perimenopause: The Prelude to Menopause

Perimenopause marks the beginning of the menopause transition. It's a phase that can start as early as a woman's late 30s or as late as her 50s, typically lasting around four to eight years. During perimenopause, the ovaries gradually start to produce less estrogen, setting off a range of changes in the body. One of the first signs that a woman is entering this phase is a change in her menstrual cycle. Periods may become irregular – they can be longer or shorter, lighter or heavier, or more or less frequent. It's a period marked by unpredictability, as the body begins its gradual shift towards menopause.

Women in perimenopause might also start experiencing some of the symptoms commonly associated with menopause, such as hot flashes, night sweats, sleep disturbances, and mood swings. These symptoms occur due to the fluctuations in hormone levels and can vary greatly in intensity and frequency from woman to woman.

Menopause: The End of Reproductive Years

Menopause is defined retrospectively after a woman has gone 12 consecutive months without a menstrual period. On average, women reach menopause around the age of 51, though this can vary widely. This stage signifies the end of the reproductive years, marked by the ovaries ceasing to release eggs and the end of menstrual cycles.

The hallmark of menopause is the significant drop in estrogen levels, which can lead to various symptoms like those experienced in perimenopause but often more intensified. Some women might also experience new symptoms, such as vaginal dryness, decreased libido, and urinary issues. The intensity and duration of these symptoms can vary; for some, they may be brief and mild, while for others, they can be more severe and persist for several years.

Postmenopause: Life After Menopause

Postmenopause is the period following menopause, marking the beginning of a new phase in a woman's life. Once a woman has reached postmenopause, her estrogen levels will have significantly decreased, and she will no longer have menstrual periods. The symptoms of menopause, like hot flashes and night sweats, often diminish in this stage, but the decrease in estrogen brings new health considerations.

One of the major concerns in postmenopause is the increased risk of osteoporosis. Estrogen plays a crucial role in maintaining bone density, and its reduced levels can lead to bones becoming weaker and more prone to fractures. Another significant concern is the increased risk of cardiovascular disease, as estrogen's protective effects on the heart and blood vessels diminish.

Navigating Each Stage

Understanding what to expect in each stage of menopause can help women better prepare and manage the transition.

In Perimenopause

Monitoring Menstrual Changes: Keeping track of menstrual cycle changes can help in identifying the onset of perimenopause.

Managing Symptoms: Adopting lifestyle changes, such as a healthy diet, regular exercise, and stress management techniques, can help alleviate the symptoms.

During Menopause

Seeking Medical Advice: Consulting with a healthcare provider can help manage more severe symptoms. Options such as hormone replacement therapy (HRT) can be considered, depending on individual health needs and risk factors.

Emotional Support: This is a time when emotional support from family, friends, or support groups can be particularly valuable.

In Postmenopause

Focus on Long-Term Health: Regular health screenings, including bone density tests, mammograms, and cardiovascular health checks, are essential.

Lifestyle Adjustments: Continuing with a healthy lifestyle is crucial. This includes maintaining a balanced diet rich in calcium and vitamin D, engaging in weight-bearing exercises to strengthen bones, and regular aerobic exercise to support heart health.

Embracing the Menopause Journey

The journey through menopause is a unique experience for every woman. While it can be challenging, it's also an opportunity for growth and new beginnings. Understanding the stages of menopause – perimenopause, menopause, and postmenopause – and their respective challenges and opportunities can empower women to navigate this transition with confidence and positivity. With the right information, support, and care, the menopause journey can be a time of empowerment and renewal, opening the door to a fulfilling and healthy post-reproductive phase of life.

How Menopause Affects Different Body Systems

Menopause, often discussed in the context of its most noticeable symptoms like hot flashes and mood swings, actually has far-reaching effects on various body systems. This natural phase in a woman's life, marking the end of her reproductive years, brings with it changes that can impact everything from bone health to cardiovascular function. In this blog, we explore how menopause affects different body systems, shedding light on the broad scope of this significant life transition.

The Cardiovascular System

One of the most critical changes during menopause concerns the cardiovascular system. Estrogen, which declines during menopause, is believed to have a protective effect on the heart and blood vessels. Its reduction is associated with an increased risk of developing cardiovascular diseases. As estrogen levels decrease, women might experience changes in their cholesterol levels, with an increase in LDL (bad cholesterol) and a decrease in HDL (good cholesterol). Additionally, the blood vessels may become less flexible, leading to a higher risk of hypertension and other heart-related conditions.

The Skeletal System

Another significant impact of menopause is on the skeletal system, particularly concerning bone density. Estrogen plays a vital role in maintaining bone strength and density. With its decrease, the process of bone resorption (breaking down of bone tissue) can outpace the formation of new bone, leading to an increased risk of osteoporosis. Osteoporosis makes bones more fragile and prone to fractures, particularly in the hip, spine, and wrist.

The Reproductive System

The most well-known effect of menopause is on the reproductive system. The ovaries cease producing eggs, and menstrual cycles come to an end. Additionally, decreased estrogen levels lead to changes in the vagina, such as dryness, thinning of the vaginal walls, and decreased elasticity, often resulting in discomfort during intercourse and increased vulnerability to vaginal infections.

The Urinary System

Menopause also affects the urinary system. The urethra can become dry, inflamed, or irritated due to the decrease in estrogen. This change can lead to an increased frequency of urination and a higher risk of urinary tract infections. Some women may also experience urinary incontinence due to the weakening of the pelvic floor muscles that occurs with age and hormonal changes.

The Endocrine System

The endocrine system, which includes glands that produce hormones, undergoes significant changes during menopause. With the ovaries producing less estrogen and progesterone, there can be effects on other hormones as well. For instance, some women may experience thyroid issues during menopause, as hormonal fluctuations can impact thyroid function.

The Nervous System

Menopause can also affect the nervous system. Fluctuations in hormone levels can influence mood, memory, and cognitive functions. Many women report experiencing mood swings, anxiety, and depression during menopause. Additionally, some may notice a decrease in concentration and memory, often referred to as "menopausal fog."

The Integumentary System

The integumentary system, which includes the skin, hair, and nails, also feels the effects of menopause. As estrogen levels decline, the skin can become thinner, less elastic, and more prone to wrinkling. There might also be changes in hair texture and an increase in hair loss or thinning.

The Digestive System

Though less directly linked, menopause can impact the digestive system as well. Hormonal changes can affect metabolism, often leading to weight gain, particularly around the abdomen. Some women also report experiencing bloating, indigestion, and changes in bowel habits during this time.

Lifestyle and Management

Understanding how menopause affects different body systems highlights the importance of a holistic approach to health during this phase. Adopting a healthy lifestyle becomes even more crucial. Regular exercise, particularly weight-bearing and cardiovascular workouts, can help maintain bone density and heart health. A balanced diet rich in calcium, vitamin D, and fiber supports bone, digestive, and overall health. It's also essential to manage stress and prioritize mental health, as psychological well-being is deeply intertwined with physical health.

Regular check-ups and health screenings are vital to monitor changes and address any issues early on. For symptoms that significantly impact quality of life, various treatments, including hormone replacement therapy (HRT), non-hormonal therapies, and natural remedies, can be explored under the guidance of a healthcare professional.

Conclusion

Menopause is a complex process that affects more than just the reproductive system. It brings changes that can touch every aspect of a woman's health. By understanding these changes and taking proactive steps to manage them, women can navigate this transition more effectively. Embracing menopause as a natural part of aging and focusing on holistic well-being can lead to a healthy and fulfilling post-menopausal life.

Chapter 3: Common Symptoms and Their Causes

Physical Symptoms: Hot Flashes, Night Sweats, Sleep Disturbances, Weight Gain

Menopause, a natural phase in a woman's life, is often synonymous with its most talked-about symptoms–hot flashes, night sweats, sleep disturbances, and weight gain. These symptoms are not just physical discomforts; they significantly affect a woman's daily life, well-being, and overall health. This blog post delves into these common physical symptoms of menopause, exploring their causes, impacts, and management strategies.

Hot Flashes: The Heat Wave

Hot flashes are perhaps the most emblematic symptom of menopause. A hot flash is a sudden feeling of warmth that spreads over the body, creating a flush or redness, particularly noticeable on the face and upper body. Some women may also experience sweating and a rapid heartbeat. Hot flashes can range in intensity and frequency, with some women experiencing them a few times a week and others several times a day. They are caused by the hormonal changes in the body that affect the brain's regulation of temperature.

The unpredictability of hot flashes can be challenging. They can occur at any time, often without warning, disrupting daily activities or sleep. While they are not harmful, their frequency and intensity can be uncomfortable and, at times, embarrassing, especially when they occur in social or professional settings.

Night Sweats: Disruptions in the Dark

Closely related to hot flashes are night sweats, which are essentially hot flashes that occur during sleep. They can be so intense that they soak nightclothes and bedding, significantly disrupting sleep. The loss of estrogen affects the hypothalamus–the body's temperature control center–causing it to falsely detect an increase in body temperature and respond by releasing heat.

Sleep disturbances caused by night sweats can lead to chronic sleep deprivation, resulting in fatigue, irritability, and difficulty concentrating. Consistently poor sleep can also have long-term health consequences, including an increased risk for cardiovascular diseases and obesity.

Sleep Disturbances: The Restless Nights

Apart from night sweats, menopause can bring other sleep disturbances, such as insomnia, restless sleep, and frequent awakenings. Fluctuations in hormone levels, particularly progesterone, which is known to have a sleep-inducing effect, contribute to these sleep issues. Stress and anxiety, common during menopause, can further exacerbate sleep difficulties.

Quality sleep is essential for good health, and its deprivation can affect mood, cognitive function, and physical health. Chronic sleep disturbances have been linked to a higher risk of developing depression, anxiety, and other health issues.

Weight Gain: The Unwelcome Change

Many women find that they gain weight during menopause, particularly around the abdomen. This weight gain can be attributed to a combination of factors, including hormonal changes, aging, lifestyle, and genetics. The decrease in estrogen levels can lead to a lower metabolic rate, while the natural aging process leads to a loss of muscle mass and a subsequent decrease in how many calories the body burns at rest.

Weight gain during menopause is not just a cosmetic concern. It can increase the risk of several health issues, including heart disease, diabetes, and certain types of cancer. Managing this weight gain through diet and exercise is crucial, but it can be challenging due to the other changes occurring in the body.

Managing Menopause Symptoms

While these symptoms might seem daunting, there are several ways to manage them effectively.

Lifestyle Changes

Adopting a healthy lifestyle can significantly mitigate menopause symptoms. Regular physical activity, especially cardiovascular and weight-bearing exercises, can help manage weight, improve sleep, and reduce the severity of hot flashes. A balanced diet rich in fruits, vegetables, whole grains, and lean proteins can support overall health and help regulate weight.

Stress Reduction

Practices such as yoga, meditation, and deep breathing can reduce stress levels, improving sleep quality and overall well-being. Finding time for hobbies and activities that bring joy can also be a good way to reduce stress.

Medical Interventions

For some women, lifestyle changes alone may not be enough to manage their symptoms effectively. In such cases, medical interventions like hormone replacement therapy (HRT) or other medications can be beneficial. It's important to discuss these options with a healthcare provider to understand the benefits and risks.

Conclusion

The physical symptoms of menopause – hot flashes, night sweats, sleep disturbances, and weight gain – are more than just inconveniences; they can significantly impact a woman's life. However, understanding these symptoms, their causes, and effective management strategies can help mitigate their impact. By focusing on a healthy lifestyle, stress reduction techniques, and seeking medical advice when necessary, women can navigate through menopause more comfortably and maintain their quality of life.

Emotional and Mental Health Symptoms: Mood Swings, Depression, Anxiety

Menopause, commonly characterized by its physical symptoms, also has profound impacts on emotional and mental health. Women going through menopause often experience mood swings, depression, and anxiety, which can be as challenging as the physical changes. This blog post aims to explore these emotional and mental health symptoms associated with menopause, their causes, and ways to manage them.

Understanding the Emotional Rollercoaster of Menopause

The transition into menopause is a significant life change that can trigger a variety of emotional responses. Fluctuating hormone levels directly affect the brain and can lead to mood swings, depression, and anxiety. These symptoms can be bewildering and unsettling, significantly impacting daily life and overall well-being.

Mood Swings: The Emotional Ups and Downs

Mood swings during menopause are characterized by rapid changes in emotion – one moment feeling content, and suddenly feeling irritable or sad without any apparent reason. These mood fluctuations can be attributed to the hormonal changes, especially the decrease in estrogen, which plays a key role in regulating mood. Estrogen interacts with chemicals in the brain that affect mood, such as serotonin and dopamine. As the levels of estrogen fluctuate and eventually decline, these mood-regulating chemicals also get affected, leading to mood swings.

Women may find themselves reacting more emotionally or unpredictably than usual. These mood swings can strain personal and professional relationships, and even the woman's own sense of self-understanding and control.

Depression: More Than Just Sadness

Menopause can also heighten the risk of depression. This is not just the occasional sadness or blues, but a persistent feeling of deep sadness, loss of interest in activities once enjoyed, feelings of worthlessness or hopelessness, and in some cases, thoughts of self-harm or suicide. While not every woman will experience depression during menopause, those with a history of depression or significant stressors are at a higher risk.

The hormonal upheavals, combined with life stressors common during the menopausal phase – like aging parents, children leaving home, or reflections on life achievements – can contribute to the onset or worsening of depressive symptoms.

Anxiety: A Heightened Sense of Worry

Anxiety during menopause often manifests as a constant or overwhelming sense of worry, nervousness, or panic about everyday situations. These feelings can be accompanied by physical symptoms such as heart palpitations, sweating, and trembling. For some women, menopause can bring on their first experiences of anxiety, while for others, it can exacerbate existing anxiety disorders.

The fluctuations in hormone levels, particularly estrogen, play a significant role in these heightened anxiety levels. Estrogen interacts with the brain's stress response system, and as its levels fluctuate, so does the response system, leading to increased feelings of anxiety.

Managing Emotional and Mental Health Symptoms

Navigating these emotional and mental health symptoms requires a multifaceted approach, combining lifestyle changes, support systems, and possibly medical interventions.

Lifestyle Adjustments

Maintaining a healthy lifestyle can have a positive impact on emotional and mental health. Regular physical exercise, particularly activities like yoga or tai chi, can reduce stress and enhance mood. A balanced diet, adequate sleep, and relaxation techniques like meditation or deep breathing exercises can also help in managing mood swings, depression, and anxiety.

Social Support and Communication

Having a strong support system is crucial. Talking openly about feelings with friends, family, or support groups can provide comfort and practical advice. Sharing experiences with others going through similar situations can be particularly reassuring.

Professional Help

For symptoms that significantly impact quality of life, seeking professional help is important. Therapists and counselors can provide strategies to manage these emotional changes. In some cases, medications such as antidepressants or anti-anxiety drugs, prescribed by a healthcare professional, can be beneficial.

Mindfulness and Cognitive Behavioral Therapy (CBT)

Practices such as mindfulness and therapies like CBT can be effective in managing mood swings and anxiety. These techniques focus on altering negative thought patterns and developing coping strategies to deal with emotional challenges.

Conclusion

The emotional and mental health symptoms of menopause – mood swings, depression, and anxiety – are significant and deserve as much attention as the physical symptoms. Understanding these symptoms and their causes is the first step towards managing them effectively. By focusing on a healthy lifestyle, seeking support, and getting professional help when necessary, women can navigate through menopause more comfortably. Acknowledging and addressing these symptoms can lead to a better quality of life and a more positive menopause experience.

Long-term Health Considerations: Osteoporosis, Heart Health

Menopause, while a natural and inevitable phase in a woman's life, ushers in changes that extend beyond the immediate symptoms of hot flashes and mood swings. Two of the most significant long-term health considerations for women post-menopause are osteoporosis and heart health. This blog post will delve into these concerns, understanding their connection with menopause, and discussing ways to manage and mitigate the risks.

Osteoporosis: Understanding the Bone Health Challenge

Osteoporosis, characterized by weakened bones that are more susceptible to fractures, is a major concern for post-menopausal women. Estrogen, a hormone that declines during menopause, plays a vital role in maintaining bone density. It helps in the absorption of calcium and other minerals essential for bone health. With the decrease in estrogen levels during and after menopause, the process of bone remodeling is affected, leading to an accelerated loss of bone density. This loss increases the risk of osteoporosis and makes bones more brittle and prone to fractures, especially in the hip, spine, and wrist.

The challenge with osteoporosis is that it is often a 'silent' condition, going undetected until a fracture occurs. This makes prevention and early detection crucial. Regular bone density screenings, especially for those with risk factors such as a family history of osteoporosis, smoking, or a history of bone fractures, are important for early intervention.

Heart Health: The Menopausal Impact

The risk of cardiovascular disease increases for women after menopause. Estrogen is believed to have a protective effect on heart health, aiding in the maintenance of flexible arteries and healthy cholesterol levels. As estrogen levels drop during menopause, women face an increased risk of developing cardiovascular conditions such as heart disease and stroke.

Post-menopausal women often experience changes in their lipid profiles, including an increase in LDL (bad cholesterol) and a decrease in HDL (good cholesterol). Additionally, changes in blood pressure and the development of arterial stiffness can further contribute to cardiovascular risks. These risks are compounded if other factors like obesity, a sedentary lifestyle, smoking, or a family history of heart disease are present.

Managing and Preventing Osteoporosis and Heart Disease

The management and prevention of osteoporosis and heart disease involve a combination of lifestyle changes, medical interventions, and regular health screenings.

Prioritizing Bone Health

To combat the risk of osteoporosis, calcium and vitamin D intake is essential. Calcium-rich foods, including dairy products, leafy green vegetables, and fortified foods, should be incorporated into the diet. Vitamin D, necessary for calcium absorption, can be obtained from sunlight exposure and dietary sources such as fatty fish and fortified foods. Supplements may also be recommended if dietary intake is insufficient.

Weight-bearing exercises like walking, jogging, and strength training are crucial for maintaining and building bone density. These exercises help in stimulating the bones to generate new tissue, keeping them strong and healthy.

Protecting Heart Health

For heart health, a diet low in saturated fats and high in fiber, fruits, vegetables, and whole grains is recommended. Foods rich in omega-3 fatty acids, like salmon and walnuts, are also beneficial for heart health. Regular physical activity, including aerobic exercises like swimming, cycling, and brisk walking, helps in maintaining a healthy weight, reducing blood pressure, and improving overall heart function.

Quitting smoking and moderating alcohol intake are also important steps in reducing heart disease risk. Smoking is a significant risk factor for heart diseases, and alcohol consumption should be limited to moderate levels.

Regular health screenings, including blood pressure checks, cholesterol level tests, and diabetes screenings, are important for early detection and management of potential heart issues.

Hormone Replacement Therapy (HRT)

Hormone Replacement Therapy can be an effective treatment for menopausal symptoms and has also been shown to have positive effects on bone density. However, its impact on heart health is more complex and can vary depending on the individual and the timing of initiation relative to menopause. Women considering HRT should discuss the potential benefits and risks with their healthcare provider to make an informed decision based on their personal health profile.

Conclusion

Understanding the long-term health implications of menopause, particularly osteoporosis and heart health, is crucial for post-menopausal women. By adopting a healthy lifestyle, undergoing regular health screenings, and seeking appropriate medical interventions, women can effectively manage these risks. Staying informed and proactive about health during and after menopause is key to maintaining a high quality of life in the post-menopausal years.

Chapter 4: Medical Management of Menopause

Hormone Replacement Therapy (HRT): Benefits, Risks, and Alternatives

Hormone Replacement Therapy (HRT) is one of the most discussed treatments in the context of menopause, known for its effectiveness in alleviating menopausal symptoms but also for its associated risks. In this blog post, we will delve into what HRT entails, its benefits, the risks involved, and explore the alternatives available for women going through menopause.

Understanding Hormone Replacement Therapy

HRT involves supplementing the body's natural hormones, estrogen and progesterone, which decrease during menopause. It can be administered in various forms, including pills, patches, gels, and creams. The primary goal of HRT is to relieve menopausal symptoms like hot flashes, night sweats, vaginal dryness, and to prevent bone loss that can lead to osteoporosis.

The Benefits of HRT

The most immediate benefit of HRT is the relief of menopausal symptoms. Many women find that HRT significantly reduces the frequency and severity of hot flashes and night sweats. It can also alleviate vaginal symptoms, such as dryness and discomfort during intercourse, making it an effective treatment for improving sexual health and quality of life during menopause.

HRT is also beneficial in preventing bone loss and reducing the risk of osteoporosis, a significant concern for post-menopausal women. By supplementing estrogen, HRT helps maintain bone density, thereby lowering the risk of fractures.

The Risks Associated with HRT

While HRT can be highly effective, it is not without risks. These risks can depend on various factors, including the type of HRT, the dosage, the duration of treatment, and the individual health profile of the woman.

One of the primary concerns with HRT is the increased risk of certain types of cancer. Studies have shown that HRT, especially when estrogen is taken without progesterone, can increase the risk of endometrial cancer. There is also an associated risk of breast cancer, particularly with long-term use of combined estrogen-progesterone therapies.

In addition to cancer risks, HRT may increase the likelihood of cardiovascular problems, such as heart disease, stroke, and blood clots, particularly in older women or those who start HRT several years after menopause.

Alternatives to Hormone Replacement Therapy

Given the risks associated with HRT, many women seek alternative treatments to manage menopausal symptoms. These alternatives range from lifestyle changes and natural remedies to non-hormonal medications.

Lifestyle Changes

Implementing lifestyle changes can significantly alleviate menopausal symptoms. Regular exercise, especially aerobic and weight-bearing exercises, can help manage weight, improve mood, and maintain bone health. A diet rich in calcium, vitamin D, and phytoestrogens (plant estrogens found in soy and flaxseeds) can also be beneficial. Additionally, avoiding triggers like hot drinks, spicy food, and alcohol can reduce the frequency of hot flashes.

Non-Hormonal Medications

For women who cannot or choose not to use HRT, non-hormonal medications can provide relief. Certain antidepressants, like SSRIs and SNRIs, can reduce hot flashes and help with mood swings. Other medications, like gabapentin, commonly used for nerve pain, have also been effective in treating hot flashes.

Natural Remedies

Natural remedies, including herbal supplements like black cohosh, red clover, and evening primrose oil, are popular among menopausal women. While some women find these remedies helpful, it's important to approach them with caution as the scientific evidence supporting their effectiveness is mixed, and they can interact with other medications.

Mind-Body Practices

Mind-body practices such as yoga, tai chi, and meditation can be effective in reducing stress and improving overall well-being. These practices can help manage the psychological symptoms of menopause, such as anxiety and mood swings.

Making an Informed Decision

Deciding whether to use HRT is a personal choice that should be made after careful consideration of the benefits and risks. It's essential for women to discuss their individual health profiles, concerns, and treatment options with their healthcare providers. This decision-making process should involve considering personal health history, family history, and the severity of menopausal symptoms.

Conclusion

Hormone Replacement Therapy remains a highly effective treatment for menopausal symptoms but comes with certain risks that must be carefully weighed. For those seeking alternatives, a range of options from lifestyle modifications to non-hormonal medications and natural remedies are available. The key to managing menopause effectively lies in staying informed, discussing options with healthcare providers, and choosing a path that aligns with one's personal health needs and lifestyle preferences. By taking a proactive approach, women can navigate menopause more comfortably and maintain their quality of life.

Non-Hormonal Medical Treatments

While Hormone Replacement Therapy (HRT) is a widely known treatment for menopause symptoms, it is not suitable for all women. Various non-hormonal medical treatments can effectively alleviate many of the discomforts associated with menopause. These treatments range from prescription medications to over-the-counter remedies, providing alternative options for those who cannot or choose not to use HRT. In this blog post, we will explore the various non-hormonal medical treatments available for managing menopause symptoms.

Understanding Non-Hormonal Treatments

Non-hormonal treatments offer relief from menopause symptoms without the use of estrogen or progesterone. These alternatives can be particularly beneficial for women with specific health concerns, such as a history of breast cancer, heart disease, or those at risk of blood clots, where HRT might not be advisable.

Antidepressants for Mood and Hot Flashes

Antidepressants, especially Selective Serotonin Reuptake Inhibitors (SSRIs) and Serotonin-Norepinephrine Reuptake Inhibitors (SNRIs), have been found to be effective in treating hot flashes. These medications can alleviate the frequency and severity of hot flashes and also help with mood swings, anxiety, and depression, which are common during menopause. Drugs like Venlafaxine, Fluoxetine, and Paroxetine are often prescribed for their dual benefits on mood and hot flashes. It is important to note that while these medications can be helpful, they come with their own set of potential side effects, such as nausea, weight gain, and sexual dysfunction.

Gabapentin for Hot Flashes

Originally used for treating seizures, Gabapentin has been found to be effective in reducing hot flashes. It can be particularly helpful for women who experience hot flashes at night and have difficulties with sleep. Gabapentin works by affecting the electrical activity in the brain and the way nerves send messages to the brain. Some women might experience side effects like dizziness, fatigue, and headaches, but many find it a useful alternative to hormonal treatments.

Clonidine for Hot Flashes

Clonidine, a medication primarily used to treat high blood pressure, can also provide relief from hot flashes. Available in pill form or as a patch, Clonidine works by affecting the blood vessels and reducing their activity. While it can be a suitable option for those unable to use HRT or other treatments, common side effects include dry mouth, drowsiness, and dizziness.

Vaginal Moisturizers and Lubricants

For vaginal dryness, a common menopause symptom, non-hormonal vaginal moisturizers and lubricants can be effective. Vaginal moisturizers are long-lasting and designed to help with overall vaginal dryness, while lubricants are used primarily to reduce discomfort during intercourse. These products are generally safe, widely available, and can be used as needed without a prescription.

Cognitive Behavioral Therapy (CBT)

CBT, a type of psychotherapy, has been effective in managing mood swings, depression, and anxiety during menopause. It helps women identify and change negative thought patterns and behaviors that cause or worsen sleep problems with habits that promote sound sleep.

Mind-Body Practices

Mind-body practices such as yoga, tai chi, and meditation can be beneficial for overall well-being during menopause. These practices can reduce stress, improve mood, and enhance sleep quality. Yoga and tai chi combine physical postures with breathing exercises and meditation, which can be particularly helpful in managing mood swings and improving sleep. Meditation focuses on breathing and awareness to reduce stress and improve mental well-being.

Dietary Supplements

Certain dietary supplements are popular for their potential to alleviate menopausal symptoms, though their effectiveness and safety can vary.

Phytoestrogens

Phytoestrogens are plant-based estrogens found in foods like soy, flaxseed, and legumes. They may help with mild hot flashes but should be used with caution, particularly in women with a history of breast cancer or other hormone-sensitive conditions.

Black Cohosh and Other Herbal Supplements

Black Cohosh is often used for hot flashes and mood swings. While some women find relief with this supplement, the evidence on its effectiveness is mixed, and there are concerns about liver health. It's important to approach herbal remedies with caution and under the guidance of a healthcare professional.

Lifestyle Modifications

Lifestyle changes are an integral part of managing menopause symptoms effectively. A healthy diet and regular exercise can alleviate some menopausal symptoms and improve overall health. Stress reduction techniques like yoga, meditation, and mindfulness can help in managing mood swings and improving sleep quality.

Conclusion

Non-hormonal medical treatments offer a range of options for managing menopause symptoms effectively without the use of hormone replacement therapy. From medications like antidepressants and Gabapentin to lifestyle changes and mind-body practices, these alternatives can be tailored to suit individual needs and preferences. It is important to discuss these options with a healthcare provider

Understanding and Navigating Healthcare for Menopause

Navigating the healthcare landscape during menopause can be daunting. With a range of symptoms affecting various aspects of health and well-being, understanding how to access and utilize healthcare services effectively is crucial. This blog post aims to guide women through the complexities of seeking and receiving healthcare during menopause, ensuring they get the support and treatment they need during this significant life stage.

Recognizing the Need for Professional Help

The first step in effectively managing menopause is recognizing when it's time to seek professional medical advice. Symptoms of menopause can vary widely among women, but certain signs indicate the need for a healthcare provider's input. Persistent or severe symptoms that interfere with daily life, such as intense hot flashes, severe mood swings, significant sleep disturbances, and concerns about long-term health risks like osteoporosis, are all valid reasons to consult a healthcare professional.

Choosing the Right Healthcare Provider

Finding a healthcare provider who is knowledgeable about menopause is critical. This might be a gynecologist, a primary care physician, or even a menopause specialist. The right provider should be someone with whom you feel comfortable discussing personal issues and who has the expertise to provide the necessary care and advice.

Gynecologists and Primary Care Physicians

Gynecologists specialize in women's reproductive health and are typically well-versed in menopause management. Primary care physicians can also provide guidance and, if needed, referrals to specialists. The key is to choose a provider who listens, understands, and takes your concerns seriously.

Menopause Specialists

In some cases, consulting a menopause specialist may be beneficial, especially for complex or severe symptoms. These specialists have in-depth knowledge of menopause and can offer a comprehensive approach to managing its various aspects.

Preparing for Healthcare Visits

To make the most of your healthcare visits, being prepared is essential. This means gathering relevant information, such as details of your menstrual cycle, a list of symptoms and how they're affecting your life, and any medical history that could be relevant to your menopause experience. It's also helpful to have a list of questions or concerns to discuss during the appointment, ensuring you don't forget to address any key points.

Effective Communication with Healthcare Providers

Effective communication is crucial in ensuring you get the best possible care. This involves being open and honest about your symptoms, concerns, and lifestyle. It's important to describe your symptoms in detail, including their frequency, severity, and impact on your daily life. If you're considering treatments like hormone replacement therapy, it's crucial to discuss the potential benefits and risks with your healthcare provider.

Advocating for Yourself

Advocating for yourself is an essential part of navigating healthcare for menopause. This means speaking up about your concerns, asking questions if something is unclear, and even seeking a second opinion if you're not comfortable with the advice or treatment plan provided. Remember, you have the right to comprehensive and respectful care.

Understanding Treatment Options

Menopause can be managed through various treatment options, ranging from lifestyle adjustments and hormone replacement therapy to non-hormonal medications and alternative therapies. Understanding these options, their benefits, and potential risks is crucial in making informed decisions about your care.

Utilizing Resources and Support

In addition to healthcare providers, there are other resources and forms of support available. These include menopause support groups, educational resources like books and reputable websites, and even online forums. Connecting with others going through similar experiences can provide valuable insights and emotional support.

Embracing a Holistic Approach

Managing menopause effectively often requires a holistic approach. This means not only addressing the physical symptoms but also considering the emotional and psychological aspects. Practices like yoga, meditation, and mindfulness can be beneficial in managing stress and improving overall well-being.

Navigating Insurance and Healthcare Systems

Understanding your insurance coverage and the healthcare system is crucial in accessing the care you need. This might involve understanding what services are covered, how to get referrals to specialists, and what out-of-pocket costs may be involved. Don't hesitate to contact your insurance provider for clarification on your coverage.

Conclusion

Navigating healthcare for menopause requires an understanding of when to seek help, how to choose the right healthcare provider, and how to advocate for yourself. By preparing for healthcare visits, communicating effectively with providers, and utilizing available resources and support, women can navigate this transition more effectively. Embracing a holistic approach to care, understanding treatment options, and navigating the healthcare system are all key to ensuring a positive menopause experience.

Chapter 5: Lifestyle Approaches to Managing Symptoms

Diet and Nutrition: Foods to Favor and Avoid

Navigating menopause often involves addressing changes in metabolism, energy levels, and overall health, which makes diet and nutrition key components of managing this life stage. The right diet can help alleviate some menopausal symptoms, maintain weight, and reduce the risk of post-menopausal health issues. In this blog, we'll explore the foods that are beneficial during menopause, as well as those best limited or avoided.

Understanding the Dietary Needs During Menopause

Menopause brings about hormonal changes that can impact bone health, cardiovascular health, and metabolism. Estrogen, which plays a role in using calcium and maintaining cholesterol levels, decreases significantly during menopause, affecting overall nutritional needs. Additionally, many women experience a slowing metabolism and changes in body composition, such as increased abdominal fat.

Foods to Favor

Phytoestrogens

Phytoestrogens are plant-derived compounds that mimic the effects of estrogen in the body. They can be found in foods like soybeans, tofu, tempeh, flaxseeds, and legumes. Including these foods in your diet may help balance hormones and reduce symptoms like hot flashes. However, it's important to consume them in moderation, especially for women with a history of hormone-sensitive conditions.

Calcium and Vitamin D for Bone Health

With an increased risk of osteoporosis during menopause, foods rich in calcium and vitamin D are crucial. Dairy products, leafy green vegetables, and calcium-fortified foods help maintain bone density. Vitamin D, essential for calcium absorption, can be obtained from the sun, fatty fish, egg yolks, and fortified foods. Supplements may also be recommended to ensure adequate intake.

Whole Grains for Heart Health

Whole grains like brown rice, quinoa, oats, and whole wheat are high in fiber, which can help manage weight, reduce cholesterol levels, and maintain digestive health. These foods also provide essential nutrients like B vitamins, magnesium, and iron, supporting overall health and energy levels.

Fruits and Vegetables

A diet rich in fruits and vegetables provides vital nutrients, antioxidants, and fiber. These foods can help manage weight, reduce the risk of chronic diseases, and support overall well-being. Aiming for a variety of colors in your fruits and vegetables ensures a broad range of nutrients.

Lean Proteins

Lean proteins such as chicken, fish, beans, and legumes are essential for maintaining muscle mass, which tends to decrease with age. They also provide satiety, which is helpful for weight management.

Healthy Fats

Incorporating healthy fats, found in olive oil, avocados, nuts, and seeds, is important for heart health and overall nutrition. Omega-3 fatty acids, particularly from fatty fish like salmon, are beneficial for reducing inflammation and supporting brain and heart health.

Foods to Limit or Avoid

High-Fat and High-Sugar Foods

Foods high in saturated fats and sugars can contribute to weight gain and increase the risk of heart disease. Processed foods, sugary snacks, and baked goods should be consumed in moderation.

Spicy Foods

For some women, spicy foods can trigger hot flashes. Monitoring how your body reacts to spicy foods and adjusting your diet accordingly can help manage this symptom.

Caffeine and Alcohol

Caffeine and alcohol can affect sleep quality and trigger hot flashes in some women. Reducing intake, especially in the evening, can improve sleep and overall symptom management.

Excessive Salt

High salt intake can contribute to increased blood pressure, a concern for heart health during menopause. Limiting processed and canned foods, which often contain high levels of sodium, is advisable.

Balancing Macronutrients

A balanced intake of carbohydrates, proteins, and fats is crucial for overall health, especially during menopause. Opting for complex carbohydrates, diverse sources of protein, and focusing on unsaturated fats helps maintain energy levels, support metabolic health, and contribute to a feeling of well-being.

Hydration

Staying well-hydrated is essential, as water plays a role in nearly every bodily function. Adequate water intake helps in digestion, nutrient absorption, and maintaining skin health. Herbal teas can be a soothing, low-caffeine alternative for hydration.

Conclusion

Adopting a balanced diet during menopause is crucial for managing symptoms and preventing long-term health issues. By favoring nutrient-rich foods like phytoestrogens, calcium, and vitamin D sources, whole grains, fruits and vegetables, lean proteins, and healthy fats, and limiting intake of processed, high-fat, and high-sugar foods, women can navigate menopause more effectively. Paying attention to hydration and the balance of macronutrients is key to a healthy menopause journey. With the right dietary approach, this stage of life can be a time of positive health and vitality.

Exercise and Physical Activity Recommendations

Menopause is a time of significant change in a woman's life, and while it brings its unique challenges, it also presents an opportunity to focus more on personal health and well-being. Regular exercise and physical activity play a crucial role in managing menopause symptoms and reducing the risk of post-menopausal health issues. This blog post explores the types of exercises recommended for menopausal women and how they contribute to overall health and well-being.

The Importance of Exercise During Menopause

Physical activity is essential during menopause for several reasons. First, it helps in managing menopause-related symptoms such as weight gain, mood swings, and sleep disturbances. Exercise also plays a vital role in reducing the risk of chronic diseases that become more prevalent post-menopause, including osteoporosis, heart disease, and diabetes. Additionally, it can improve mental health, reducing the risk of depression and anxiety, which can be heightened during this life stage.

Cardiovascular Exercise for Heart Health

Cardiovascular or aerobic exercises are crucial for maintaining a healthy heart and improving overall fitness. Activities like brisk walking, jogging, swimming, cycling, and dancing increase heart rate and lung capacity, which is vital for cardiovascular health. As estrogen levels, which have a protective effect on the heart, decline during menopause, maintaining heart health becomes even more important.

Regular cardiovascular exercise helps in managing weight, reducing the risk of heart disease, and improving mood and energy levels. The general recommendation is to aim for at least 150 minutes of moderate-intensity aerobic activity or 75 minutes of vigorous-intensity activity per week.

Strength Training for Bone Health and Muscle Mass

Strength training or resistance exercises are particularly important during and after menopause. These exercises help in building muscle mass, which naturally decreases with age, and maintaining bone density, thereby reducing the risk of osteoporosis. Activities can include lifting weights, using resistance bands, or body-weight exercises like push-ups and squats.

Incorporating strength training into your exercise routine at least two days a week can enhance muscle strength, improve metabolism, and support posture and balance. It's also beneficial in managing weight, as increased muscle mass helps in burning more calories even at rest.

Flexibility and Balance Exercises

Exercises that focus on flexibility and balance are essential, especially as we age. Yoga and Pilates are excellent for enhancing flexibility, reducing muscle tension, and improving overall balance and posture. These practices also offer mental health benefits, including stress reduction and improved focus and mindfulness.

Balance exercises, such as tai chi or simple activities like standing on one foot or walking heel-to-toe, are important for preventing falls, which become a higher risk due to weakened bones post-menopause. Including flexibility and balance activities in your exercise routine several times a week can have long-term benefits for both physical and mental health.

The Role of Exercise in Weight Management

Weight management becomes a significant concern during menopause due to hormonal changes that can slow down metabolism and lead to weight gain, particularly around the abdomen. A combination of cardiovascular and strength-training exercises is the most effective approach to managing weight. Regular physical activity helps in burning calories, building muscle mass, and improving metabolic health.

Mental Health Benefits of Exercise

Exercise is not just beneficial for physical health; it's also crucial for mental well-being. Physical activity releases endorphins, which are natural mood lifters. It can also serve as a form of meditation, helping to clear the mind and reduce stress. Aerobic exercises, in particular, have been shown to reduce symptoms of depression and anxiety.

Exercise Tips for Menopausal Women

- **Start Slowly:** If you're new to exercise, start slowly and gradually increase intensity and duration.
- **Consistency:** Regularity is key. Find activities you enjoy to ensure you stay consistent with your exercise routine.

- **Listen to Your Body:** Pay attention to how your body responds to different types of exercises and adjust accordingly.
- **Stay Hydrated:** Drink plenty of water before, during, and after exercise, especially if experiencing hot flashes.
- **Dress Comfortably:** Wear breathable, moisture-wicking clothes to stay comfortable during exercise.

Conclusion

Incorporating regular exercise into your routine during menopause is crucial for managing symptoms, improving overall health, and maintaining a high quality of life. By focusing on a mix of cardiovascular, strength, flexibility, and balance exercises, women can effectively navigate the physical and mental challenges of menopause. Regular physical activity not only helps in managing menopause symptoms but also sets a foundation for a healthy and active post-menopausal life.

Sleep Hygiene and Stress Reduction Techniques

Menopause can significantly impact a woman's sleep and stress levels. Fluctuations in hormone levels can lead to sleep disturbances, while the physical and emotional changes associated with menopause can increase stress. In this blog, we will explore effective sleep hygiene practices and stress reduction techniques that can help manage these challenges during menopause.

The Importance of Sleep Hygiene During Menopause

Good sleep hygiene refers to the habits and practices conducive to achieving consistent, quality sleep. This is particularly important during menopause, as many women experience sleep disturbances such as insomnia, restless sleep, and night sweats. Quality sleep is crucial for overall health, including emotional well-being, cognitive function, and physical health.

Creating a Restful Sleep Environment

A comfortable and conducive sleep environment is key to improving sleep quality. This includes ensuring the bedroom is quiet, dark, and cool. Investing in comfortable bedding and using blackout curtains or eye masks to block out light can make a significant difference. Additionally, maintaining a cool room temperature can help manage night sweats, a common menopause symptom.

Establishing a Regular Sleep Routine

Consistency is crucial for good sleep hygiene. Going to bed and waking up at the same time every day, including weekends, can help regulate the body's internal clock. Developing a relaxing bedtime routine, such as reading, taking a warm bath, or practicing relaxation techniques, can signal to the body that it's time to wind down and prepare for sleep.

Managing Diet and Exercise

Diet and exercise play a significant role in sleep quality. Avoiding heavy meals, caffeine, and alcohol close to bedtime can prevent sleep disturbances. While regular exercise during the day can promote better sleep, it's best to avoid vigorous activities close to bedtime as they can be stimulating.

Reducing Stress for Better Sleep

Stress and sleep are closely linked, and managing stress is an essential part of improving sleep quality. Practices such as deep breathing, meditation, or yoga can help calm the mind and body, making it easier to fall and stay asleep.

Mindfulness and Relaxation Techniques

Mindfulness and relaxation techniques can be effective in reducing stress and improving sleep. Mindfulness involves focusing on the present moment and accepting it without judgment, which can help alleviate worry and anxiety. Techniques like progressive muscle relaxation, which involves tensing and then relaxing different muscle groups, can also promote relaxation and sleep.

Cognitive Behavioral Therapy (CBT) for Insomnia

CBT for insomnia is a structured program that helps identify and replace thoughts and behaviors that cause or worsen sleep problems with habits that promote sound sleep. It can be particularly beneficial for menopausal women experiencing sleep disturbances.

The Role of Stress Management in Menopause

Effectively managing stress is crucial during menopause. Elevated stress levels can exacerbate menopausal symptoms like hot flashes and mood swings and negatively impact sleep.

Exercise as a Stress Reliever

Regular physical activity is a powerful stress reliever. Activities like walking, swimming, or cycling can boost endorphin levels, the body's natural mood elevators, and provide a distraction from daily stressors.

Engaging in Hobbies and Activities

Engaging in hobbies or activities that bring joy and relaxation can also help reduce stress. Whether it's gardening, painting, reading, or listening to music, activities that you enjoy can be a great way to unwind and de-stress.

Seeking Social Support

Having a strong support system is important for managing stress. Talking with friends, family, or joining a support group can provide an outlet for sharing experiences and feelings, which can be a significant stress reliever.

Practicing Good Sleep Hygiene and Stress Management

Practicing good sleep hygiene and stress management involves a combination of creating the right sleep environment, establishing routines, managing diet and exercise, and incorporating stress-reducing activities and relaxation techniques. It's also about recognizing when it's time to seek professional help, whether it's for sleep disturbances or managing stress.

Conclusion

Sleep disturbances and elevated stress levels are common challenges during menopause, but with effective sleep hygiene practices and stress reduction techniques, they can be managed. Creating a conducive sleep environment, establishing a regular sleep routine, managing diet and exercise, and practicing relaxation techniques can all contribute to better sleep and reduced stress. Incorporating regular physical activity, engaging in enjoyable activities, and seeking social support are also important aspects of managing stress during menopause. By prioritizing sleep and stress management, menopausal women can improve their overall quality of life.

Chapter 6: Holistic and Alternative Therapies

Herbal Remedies and Supplements

As women navigate the often challenging waters of menopause, many turn to herbal remedies and supplements in search of natural relief from symptoms. These alternative treatments can offer benefits, but it's essential to approach them with an informed and cautious perspective. This blog explores various herbal remedies and supplements commonly used for menopause, their potential benefits, and considerations for their use.

The Allure of Herbal Remedies and Supplements

The appeal of herbal remedies and supplements lies in their natural origin and the perception that they offer a gentler, more holistic approach to managing menopause symptoms compared to conventional hormone replacement therapy (HRT). Many women seek these alternatives to avoid the potential side effects and risks associated with HRT or when HRT is not recommended due to personal health risks.

Phytoestrogens: Mimicking Estrogen

Phytoestrogens are plant-derived compounds that have a similar structure to estrogen and can mimic some of its actions in the body. They are found in foods like soybeans, flaxseeds, and some grains and herbs. The theory is that phytoestrogens might help balance hormones and alleviate menopausal symptoms like hot flashes and night sweats. However, the effectiveness of phytoestrogens can vary, and their impact on hormone-sensitive conditions, such as breast cancer, remains a subject of ongoing research and debate.

Black Cohosh: A Popular Choice for Hot Flashes

Black cohosh is one of the most widely used herbal supplements for menopause, particularly for hot flashes and night sweats. It's believed to have estrogen-like effects on the body, though its exact mechanism is not fully understood. While some studies suggest black cohosh may be helpful in reducing menopausal symptoms, the results are mixed, and its long-term safety is not well-established. Concerns have been raised about its potential effects on the liver, emphasizing the need for caution and consultation with a healthcare provider before use.

St. John's Wort: For Mood Swings and Depression

St. John's Wort is commonly used for mild to moderate depression and may be beneficial for mood swings during menopause. It's thought to work by affecting neurotransmitters in the brain that are involved in mood regulation. However, St. John's Wort can interact with a wide range of medications, including antidepressants, birth control pills, and blood thinners, making it crucial to discuss its use with a healthcare provider.

Red Clover: Another Phytoestrogen Source

Red clover, containing isoflavones – a type of phytoestrogen – has been studied for its potential to relieve hot flashes and improve bone density. However, as with other phytoestrogen sources, the evidence is mixed, and there is some concern about its use in women with a history of hormone-sensitive cancers.

Evening Primrose Oil: For Breast Pain

Evening primrose oil is often touted for its ability to alleviate breast pain, a symptom some women experience during menopause. It's also sometimes recommended for hot flashes, though scientific support for this use is limited. Evening primrose oil is generally considered safe but can have side effects like headache and stomach upset.

Ginkgo Biloba: For Mental Clarity

Ginkgo biloba is sometimes used by menopausal women for memory and concentration issues. While known for its potential cognitive benefits, studies on its effectiveness for menopausal cognitive symptoms have yielded mixed results.

Valerian Root: For Sleep Disturbances

Valerian root is commonly used for sleep disorders and might offer benefits for menopausal women experiencing insomnia or sleep disturbances. It's believed to have a sedative effect on the brain and nervous system, although more research is needed to confirm its effectiveness and safety.

Considerations for Using Herbal Remedies and Supplements

While herbal remedies and supplements can be a valuable part of managing menopause symptoms, there are important considerations to keep in mind:

- **Consult Healthcare Providers:** It's crucial to discuss any supplements with your healthcare provider, as they can interact with medications and may not be suitable for everyone.

- **Quality and Purity:** The quality and purity of supplements can vary greatly, so it's important to choose products from reputable manufacturers.

- **Research and Evidence:** Be informed about the level of scientific evidence supporting the use of any supplement and be wary of products making unsubstantiated claims.

- **Side Effects and Risks:** Understand potential side effects and risks associated with any herbal remedy or supplement.

Conclusion

Herbal remedies and supplements offer an alternative approach to managing menopause symptoms for many women. While they can provide relief and support during this transition, it's important to use them wisely, with an understanding of their potential effects and in consultation with healthcare professionals. Balancing natural approaches with informed medical advice can help women navigate menopause safely and effectively.

Mind-Body Practices: Yoga, Meditation, Tai Chi

Menopause is not just a physical transition; it encompasses emotional and mental changes that can be significant. Mind-body practices like yoga, meditation, and tai chi offer holistic ways to navigate these changes, providing benefits that extend beyond mere symptom relief. In this blog, we explore how these practices can be particularly beneficial during the menopausal transition, helping to manage symptoms, reduce stress, and enhance overall well-being.

Yoga: Flexibility, Strength, and Balance

Yoga, an ancient practice that combines physical postures, breathing exercises, and meditation, can be particularly beneficial during menopause. It helps in maintaining flexibility, building strength, and improving balance, which are crucial as the body ages. The different poses and stretches in yoga can also help alleviate some physical symptoms of menopause, like muscle tension and joint pain.

Beyond the physical benefits, yoga is highly effective in managing stress and improving mental health. The meditative aspect of yoga encourages mindfulness and can help women dealing with mood swings, anxiety, and depression, which are common during menopause. Additionally, certain yoga poses are believed to be beneficial for specific menopausal symptoms. For instance, cooling and restorative poses can help manage hot flashes, while poses that promote relaxation can improve sleep quality.

Meditation: Calming the Mind

Meditation is another powerful tool during menopause. It involves sitting quietly and focusing the mind, which can be on a specific thought, object, or simply the process of breathing. This practice helps calm the mind, reduce stress, and improve concentration. During menopause, women often experience what is commonly referred to as 'brain fog,' a condition where they may feel less mentally sharp than usual. Meditation can help combat this by enhancing cognitive function and improving focus.

Moreover, meditation has been shown to be effective in managing emotional challenges. Regular meditation can reduce the severity of mood swings, alleviate anxiety, and promote a general sense of well-being. It can also improve sleep quality, which is often a significant concern during menopause.

Tai Chi: Gentle Movements for Overall Wellness

Tai Chi, a form of martial arts known for its gentle and flowing movements, is particularly suitable for menopausal women. It is a low-impact exercise that is easy on the joints but effective in improving balance, flexibility, and muscle strength. The slow, deliberate movements of tai chi are accompanied by deep breathing, which aids in relaxation and stress reduction.

Tai Chi has been found to be beneficial in improving bone density, which is a significant concern during and after menopause due to the increased risk of osteoporosis. Its meditative aspect can help in managing stress and anxiety, and the social aspect of practicing Tai Chi in groups can provide additional emotional support.

Integrating Mind-Body Practices Into Daily Life

Incorporating mind-body practices like yoga, meditation, and tai chi into daily life can significantly improve the menopause experience. These practices do not require specialized equipment and can be adapted to different fitness levels, making them accessible to most women.

Creating a Routine

Consistency is key when it comes to mind-body practices. Even a few minutes of meditation or a short yoga or tai chi session each day can be beneficial. It's about making these practices a regular part of your routine.

Seeking Guidance

For beginners, it can be helpful to seek guidance from qualified instructors. Many community centers, gyms, and wellness studios offer classes in yoga, meditation, and tai chi. There are also numerous online resources available, including instructional videos and apps, which can be helpful, especially for meditation.

Personalization

It's important to personalize these practices to fit your individual needs and physical capabilities. Listen to your body and adjust the practices accordingly. For example, if certain yoga poses are challenging, modifications can be made.

Mindfulness in Everyday Activities

Incorporating mindfulness into everyday activities can also be beneficial. This can be as simple as paying full attention to the task at hand, whether it's eating, walking, or even listening to someone. Mindfulness practices help keep the mind engaged in the present moment, reducing stress and improving mental clarity.

Conclusion

Mind-body practices like yoga, meditation, and tai chi offer holistic benefits that can be particularly valuable during menopause. These practices help manage physical symptoms, reduce stress, improve mental health, and enhance overall quality of life. By integrating these practices into daily routines, women can navigate the challenges of menopause more effectively, embracing this stage of life with a sense of balance and well-being.

Acupuncture and Other Complementary Therapies

Menopause, a natural part of aging, often brings a multitude of symptoms that can range from mildly annoying to significantly life-altering. While traditional medical treatments are available, many women are increasingly turning to complementary therapies like acupuncture, massage, and herbal remedies to manage their symptoms. In this blog, we delve into how acupuncture and other complementary therapies can be beneficial during menopause, offering natural and holistic alternatives for symptom management.

Acupuncture: Balancing the Body's Energy

Acupuncture, a key component of traditional Chinese medicine, involves the insertion of fine needles into specific points on the body. It is based on the belief that health is governed by the flow of energy, or Qi, in the body, and that illness or symptoms are a result of blockages or imbalances in this energy.

During menopause, acupuncture is often sought to alleviate common symptoms such as hot flashes, night sweats, mood swings, and sleep disturbances. The therapy is believed to work by stimulating the body's natural healing processes, enhancing blood flow, and affecting the nervous system. This can lead to a balance in hormone levels, reduction in inflammation, and an overall sense of well-being.

Women undergoing acupuncture often report not just a reduction in specific menopausal symptoms, but also an improvement in overall health, including better sleep, more energy, and a more stable mood.

Massage Therapy: Relief through Touch

Massage therapy, another popular complementary therapy, involves the manipulation of the body's soft tissues. During menopause, massage can be particularly beneficial in managing stress, improving circulation, and relieving muscle tension. Different types of massage, such as Swedish, deep tissue, or aromatherapy massage, offer various benefits.

Swedish massage, known for its gentle, relaxing strokes, can help reduce stress and promote relaxation, which is particularly helpful for women experiencing anxiety or sleep issues. Deep tissue massage, which works on deeper layers of muscle, can be effective for relieving chronic pain and tension, often experienced in the neck, shoulders, and back during menopause.

Herbal Remedies: Natural Symptom Management

Herbal remedies, used for centuries to treat various ailments, are commonly used by menopausal women. Herbs like black cohosh, red clover, and evening primrose oil are often sought for their potential to alleviate symptoms like hot flashes and mood swings. However, the effectiveness and safety of these herbs can vary, and it's important to use them under the guidance of a healthcare professional, as they can interact with other medications and may not be suitable for everyone.

Black cohosh, for example, is believed to have estrogen-like effects on the body and may help balance hormones, although scientific evidence on its effectiveness is mixed. Red clover, containing isoflavones, a type of phytoestrogen, has been studied for its potential to improve bone density and reduce hot flashes. Evening primrose oil is often touted for its ability to improve skin health and hormonal balance.

Tai Chi and Yoga: Gentle Movement Therapies

Tai Chi and yoga are gentle movement therapies that combine physical postures with breathing exercises and meditation. They can be especially beneficial for menopausal women in managing stress, improving flexibility and balance, and enhancing overall well-being.

Tai Chi, with its slow, flowing movements, can improve balance and flexibility, reducing the risk of falls, a concern as bones become more fragile post-menopause. Yoga, known for its wide range of postures and styles, can be tailored to individual needs, offering

benefits like muscle strengthening, stress reduction, and improved
sleep.

Mind-Body Techniques: Meditation and Relaxation

Mind-body techniques such as meditation and relaxation exercises
are crucial in managing the emotional and psychological aspects
of menopause. Practices like mindfulness meditation, guided
imagery, and progressive muscle relaxation can reduce stress,
improve mood, and enhance quality of sleep.

The Role of Nutrition and Diet

In conjunction with these therapies, nutrition and diet play a key
role in managing menopause symptoms. A diet rich in phytoestrogens, calcium, and vitamin D, along with adequate hydration, can
support overall health and alleviate certain symptoms.

Navigating Complementary Therapies

Navigating complementary therapies involves researching, consulting healthcare professionals, and understanding one's own
body and needs. It's important to approach these therapies with
an open mind but also with caution, ensuring they complement
rather than replace conventional medical advice.

Conclusion

Complementary therapies like acupuncture, massage, herbal
remedies, Tai Chi, and yoga offer holistic alternatives to manage
menopause symptoms. These therapies can provide natural relief
and support overall health and well-being during menopause.
However, it's crucial to use them thoughtfully, in consultation with
healthcare professionals, and as part of a broader approach to
health during this significant life transition. By incorporating these
therapies, women can navigate menopause more comfortably
and embrace this new phase of life with a sense of balance and
well-being.

Chapter 7: Emotional Well-being and Mental Health

Coping Strategies for Mood Swings and Mental Health Challenges

Menopause is a significant life transition that brings not just physical changes but also emotional and mental challenges. Mood swings, anxiety, and depression are common experiences during this period due to hormonal fluctuations and the various life changes that often accompany this stage. This blog post aims to provide coping strategies for managing mood swings and mental health challenges associated with menopause, helping women navigate this phase with greater ease and understanding.

Understanding the Emotional Impact of Menopause

The first step in coping with the emotional and mental health challenges of menopause is to understand their origins. Hormonal changes, particularly the reduction in estrogen, directly impact the brain's chemistry and can lead to mood swings, anxiety, and depression. These changes are often compounded by sleep disturbances, stress, and other menopausal symptoms like hot flashes.

Acknowledging and Accepting the Changes

Acknowledging and accepting these emotional fluctuations as a normal part of menopause can be empowering. Understanding that these feelings are a common and natural part of the transition can help women approach their experiences without self-judgment, allowing them to seek support and care more openly.

Developing a Support Network

Having a solid support network is essential during menopause. Talking with friends, family members, or joining support groups where experiences and coping strategies can be shared can be incredibly beneficial. Sometimes, just knowing that others are going through similar experiences can be comforting and help alleviate feelings of isolation or confusion.

Seeking Professional Help

If mood swings or mental health challenges become too overwhelming, seeking professional help is crucial. Therapists or counselors specializing in menopause or women's health can offer valuable support and strategies for managing emotional changes. In some cases, they may recommend treatments like cognitive behavioral therapy (CBT) or, if necessary, medication to help manage symptoms of depression or anxiety.

Lifestyle Adjustments for Emotional Well-being

Making certain lifestyle adjustments can significantly impact emotional health. Regular physical activity, a balanced diet, adequate sleep, and engaging in activities that bring joy and relaxation can all contribute to a more stable mood and overall sense of well-being. Exercise, in particular, is a powerful tool for managing stress and improving mood due to the release of endorphins, often referred to as feel-good hormones.

Practicing Mindfulness and Relaxation Techniques

Mindfulness and relaxation techniques can be particularly effective in managing mood swings and anxiety. Practices like meditation, deep breathing exercises, and yoga encourage a focus on the present moment and promote relaxation, helping to mitigate feelings of stress and anxiety. These practices can also improve sleep quality, which in turn can have a positive effect on mood and emotional stability.

Creating a Self-Care Routine

Developing a self-care routine that includes time for relaxation, hobbies, and activities that promote happiness is vital. Self-care isn't just about physical health; it's about nurturing emotional and mental well-being. Whether it's reading, gardening, painting, or simply taking a long bath, engaging in activities that provide a sense of calm and enjoyment is crucial.

Maintaining Social Connections

Staying socially connected is important for mental health. Maintaining friendships, participating in community activities, or volunteering can provide a sense of purpose and connection, countering feelings of isolation or loneliness that sometimes accompany menopause.

Managing Stress Effectively

Effective stress management is key to coping with mood swings and mental health challenges during menopause. Techniques such as progressive muscle relaxation, guided imagery, or spending time in nature can help reduce stress levels. Identifying stressors and learning healthy ways to cope with them, such as through problem-solving or setting boundaries, can also be beneficial.

Embracing New Challenges and Opportunities

Menopause can be a time of reflection and new opportunities. Embracing this life stage as a chance for growth and exploration, whether through new hobbies, learning opportunities, or personal development endeavors, can provide a positive focus and enhance mental well-being.

Keeping a Mood Journal

Keeping a mood journal can help women track their emotional fluctuations and identify any patterns or triggers. This awareness can be helpful in developing personalized coping strategies and in discussions with healthcare providers.

Conclusion

Coping with mood swings and mental health challenges during menopause requires a multifaceted approach. By understanding the emotional impacts of menopause, developing a support network, seeking professional help when needed, and incorporating lifestyle changes, mindfulness practices, and effective stress management techniques, women can navigate this transition more smoothly. Embracing menopause as a natural and significant life stage, and focusing on self-care and personal growth, can transform this period into a time of positive change and empowerment.

Building and Utilizing Support Systems

Navigating the journey through menopause can be a complex and often challenging experience for many women. It's a time marked by significant physical, emotional, and psychological changes. One of the most effective ways to manage this transition is by building and utilizing a strong support system. This blog post will explore the importance of cultivating a network of support during menopause and how to effectively utilize these resources for a more positive menopause experience.

The Importance of a Support System During Menopause

Menopause, while a natural part of aging, often comes with a range of symptoms that can impact a woman's quality of life. These include hot flashes, sleep disturbances, mood swings, and changes in sexual health. In addition to these physical symptoms, menopause can also bring feelings of loss, anxiety about aging, and concerns about health. A strong support system can provide emotional comfort, practical advice, and a sense of understanding and solidarity.

Types of Support Systems

Support during menopause can come from various sources, each offering different types of assistance and understanding.

Family and Friends

The immediate social circle of family and friends is often the first line of support. Open communication about the experiences and challenges of menopause with family members can foster understanding and empathy. Friends, especially those who are going through or have gone through menopause, can offer valuable insights and emotional support.

Healthcare Providers

Building a relationship with healthcare providers who are knowledgeable about menopause is crucial. This can include general practitioners, gynecologists, or menopause specialists. These professionals can offer medical advice, treatment options, and guidance on managing symptoms.

Support Groups and Communities

Joining menopause support groups, whether in person or online, can connect women with others experiencing similar challenges. These groups provide a platform to share experiences, tips, and coping strategies, and can be a source of comfort and reassurance.

Professional Counseling

For some women, professional counseling can be beneficial, especially for those struggling with significant mood changes or mental health challenges. Counselors or therapists specializing in menopause can provide strategies for managing emotional and psychological changes.

Utilizing Your Support System Effectively

Having a support system in place is one thing, but utilizing it effectively is key to navigating menopause successfully.

Open Communication

Being open and honest about your experiences, needs, and feelings with your support system is crucial. This transparency allows for a deeper understanding and more meaningful support from those around you.

Seeking and Accepting Help

It's important to recognize when you need help and to be open to accepting it. Whether it's emotional support, practical help, or medical advice, reaching out and accepting assistance is a sign of strength, not weakness.

Sharing Experiences

Sharing your own experiences and listening to others can be incredibly validating and empowering. It can provide different perspectives and strategies for coping with menopause symptoms.

Staying Informed

Using your support system to stay informed about menopause and its management can be hugely beneficial. This can involve discussing the latest research and treatment options with healthcare providers or sharing information within support groups.

Balancing Support with Personal Research

While support systems are invaluable, it's also important to do your personal research and self-education about menopause. This balanced approach ensures that you are well-informed and active in your menopause management.

Emotional Support

The emotional support provided by friends, family, and support groups can be particularly beneficial during menopause. Knowing that you're not alone in your experiences can make a significant difference in how you navigate this transition.

Professional Support

Utilizing professional support, such as healthcare providers and counselors, can provide a level of expertise and guidance that is crucial for managing menopause effectively. They can offer tailored advice and treatment options based on your specific symptoms and health history.

Conclusion

Building and utilizing a support system is an essential aspect of navigating menopause. By combining the emotional and practical support from family and friends, the expertise of healthcare providers, the solidarity of support groups, and professional counseling when needed, women can face the challenges of menopause with a strong network of support. This comprehensive approach not only helps in managing the symptoms and challenges of menopause but also enhances overall well-being and quality of life during this significant life stage.

Seeking Professional Help: Therapists and Counselors

Menopause is a significant transition in a woman's life that can be accompanied by a host of physical, emotional, and psychological changes. While family and friends can provide invaluable support, there are times when the guidance of a professional therapist or counselor becomes essential. This blog post aims to explore the role of therapists and counselors in helping women navigate the challenges of menopause, highlighting the importance of seeking professional help when needed.

The Role of Therapists and Counselors in Menopause

Menopause can bring about not only physical changes but also profound emotional and psychological shifts. Hormonal fluctuations can lead to mood swings, anxiety, and depression, while the physical symptoms of menopause can significantly impact a woman's quality of life. Therapists and counselors specialize in helping individuals navigate such transitions, offering support, strategies, and a safe space to discuss feelings and experiences.

Understanding When to Seek Professional Help

Recognizing when to seek the help of a therapist or counselor is a crucial step. Signs that it might be time to seek professional help include persistent feelings of sadness, anxiety, or hopelessness; difficulties coping with daily life; significant mood swings; problems with relationships; or simply feeling overwhelmed by the experience of menopause. Seeking help is a sign of strength and an important step in taking care of one's mental health.

Types of Therapy for Menopause

Various types of therapy can be beneficial during menopause. Cognitive-behavioral therapy (CBT) is effective in helping women manage negative thoughts and behaviors that can arise during menopause. It can also be used to address specific symptoms like insomnia or anxiety. Other types of therapy, such as psychotherapy or counseling, can provide a more general approach, helping women process their experiences and develop coping strategies.

Finding the Right Therapist or Counselor

Finding a therapist or counselor who is a good fit is essential. It's important to choose a professional who has experience with menopause or women's health issues. A good therapist or counselor should be someone with whom you feel comfortable and can trust. They should provide a supportive and non-judgmental space where you can openly discuss your concerns and feelings.

The Process of Therapy

Therapy typically involves regular sessions where you discuss your experiences, feelings, and challenges. The therapist may offer insights, coping strategies, and exercises to do outside of sessions. The goal is to help you understand and manage your symptoms, develop resilience, and improve your overall well-being.

Therapy as a Space for Understanding and Growth

Menopause can be a time of reflection and personal growth. Therapy can provide the space to explore these aspects, helping you understand the changes you're going through, both physically and emotionally. It can be an opportunity to reassess life goals, relationships, and personal aspirations.

Addressing Relationship Challenges

Menopause can also affect personal relationships. Therapists and counselors can help in navigating these changes, offering strategies for communication and understanding. For some, couple's therapy may be beneficial to address changes in the relationship dynamics during menopause.

Group Therapy and Support Groups

In addition to individual therapy, group therapy or support groups can be beneficial. These groups provide a sense of community and an opportunity to share experiences with others going through similar challenges.

Teletherapy and Online Counseling Options

With advancements in technology, teletherapy and online counseling have become more accessible. These options can be particularly useful for those who have difficulty accessing in-person therapy due to location, mobility issues, or time constraints.

Integrating Therapy with Other Menopause Management Strategies

Therapy is often most effective when integrated with other menopause management strategies. This might include medical treatments, lifestyle changes, and support from family and friends. Working in conjunction with healthcare providers to create a comprehensive menopause management plan can be highly effective.

The Importance of Mental Health During Menopause

Mental health is a crucial part of overall well-being, especially during significant life transitions like menopause. Seeking the help of therapists and counselors can ensure that mental health is given the attention it deserves during this time.

Conclusion

Seeking the help of therapists and counselors can be a vital step in navigating the complexities of menopause. Professional guidance can provide support, strategies for coping, and a deeper understanding of the emotional and psychological changes occurring during this time. By acknowledging the importance of mental health and seeking appropriate support, women can navigate menopause with greater resilience and a more positive outlook.

Chapter 8: Navigating Relationships and Sexuality

Changes in Sexual Health and Libido

Menopause, a natural phase in a woman's life, brings about a variety of changes, not least of which are those related to sexual health and libido. Understanding these changes and learning how to manage them can help women maintain a fulfilling sexual life during and after the menopausal transition. This blog post aims to explore the changes in sexual health and libido that occur during menopause, their causes, and ways to manage them.

The Impact of Menopause on Sexual Health

The decline in estrogen and other hormones during menopause directly affects sexual health. Estrogen plays a crucial role in maintaining the health of the vaginal tissue, elasticity, and lubrication. As estrogen levels decrease, women may experience changes such as vaginal dryness, decreased sensation, and discomfort during sex. These physical changes can understandably lead to a decreased interest in sexual activity or a change in sexual response.

Libido and Hormonal Changes

Libido, or sexual desire, can fluctuate significantly during menopause. The hormonal changes, particularly the reduction in estrogen and testosterone, can contribute to a decreased libido. However, it's important to note that libido is influenced by a range of factors, including emotional well-being, relationship dynamics, and physical health, not just hormonal changes.

Vaginal Dryness and Discomfort

Vaginal dryness is one of the most common issues faced during menopause, leading to discomfort during intercourse. The decrease in estrogen thins the vaginal walls and reduces natural lubrication, which can make sex painful or less enjoyable. This condition, known as vaginal atrophy, can also increase the risk of vaginal infections due to changes in the vaginal pH.

Emotional Factors Affecting Sexual Health

Emotional and psychological factors can also impact sexual health during menopause. Mood swings, depression, anxiety, and stress can all contribute to a decreased interest in sex. Body image issues, stemming from other menopausal symptoms like weight gain or hot flashes, can also affect self-esteem and sexual desire.

Managing Changes in Sexual Health and Libido

Addressing the changes in sexual health and libido involves both medical and lifestyle approaches.

Lubricants and Moisturizers

For vaginal dryness, over-the-counter vaginal lubricants and moisturizers can be effective. Lubricants can be used during sexual activity to increase comfort, while moisturizers are used regularly to maintain vaginal moisture.

Hormonal Treatments

Local estrogen therapy, in the form of creams, vaginal rings, or tablets, can help alleviate vaginal dryness and discomfort. These treatments deliver estrogen directly to the vaginal tissue, helping to restore its health and lubrication.

Non-Hormonal Medications

For those who cannot or choose not to use hormonal treatments, non-hormonal medications can provide relief. Certain antidepressants, for instance, have been shown to help with hot flashes and mood swings, indirectly improving sexual health.

Communication with Partner

Open communication with a partner about the changes and challenges is crucial. Discussing what feels good, what doesn't, and exploring other forms of intimacy can help maintain a healthy sexual relationship.

Regular Sexual Activity

Maintaining regular sexual activity can improve blood flow to the genital area and help preserve vaginal health. It can also boost libido by reinforcing a routine of sexual intimacy and pleasure.

Psychological Support

Seeking psychological support for mood swings, depression, or anxiety can indirectly improve libido. Therapy, counseling, or support groups can provide tools for managing emotional changes impacting sexual health.

Lifestyle Changes

Maintaining a healthy lifestyle through diet, exercise, and stress management can improve overall well-being and sexual health. Regular exercise can boost energy levels, improve body image, and enhance mood, all of which can contribute to a healthy sex life.

Pelvic Floor Exercises

Strengthening the pelvic floor muscles through exercises such as Kegels can improve sexual sensation and orgasmic function. These exercises can also help with urinary incontinence, which is common during menopause.

Conclusion

Changes in sexual health and libido are common aspects of menopause, influenced by hormonal, physical, and psychological factors. By understanding these changes and exploring various strategies, from open communication with partners and maintaining a healthy lifestyle to seeking medical advice and psychological support, women can navigate these challenges effectively. Embracing menopause as a natural part of life and focusing on holistic well-being can lead to a satisfying and fulfilling sexual life during and after this transition.

Communicating with Partners and Family Members

Menopause is a significant life transition that not only affects women undergoing it but also impacts their relationships with partners and family members. Effective communication during this time is crucial for maintaining healthy relationships and ensuring mutual understanding and support. This blog post will discuss the importance of open communication with partners and family members about menopause, offering insights into how to navigate these conversations effectively.

The Impact of Menopause on Relationships

Menopause can bring about a range of physical and emotional changes that may affect a woman's interactions and relationships with those close to her. Symptoms like mood swings, irritability, and changes in sexual desire can create misunderstandings and tensions, especially if partners and family members are unaware or uninformed about the causes of these changes.

Opening the Lines of Communication

Starting a conversation about menopause can be challenging but is essential for fostering understanding. It's important to share what you are experiencing and how it might be affecting your behavior or mood. This conversation doesn't have to be a one-time event but rather an ongoing dialogue as you navigate through different stages and symptoms of menopause.

Discussing Physical Changes

Physical changes during menopause, such as hot flashes, sleep disturbances, or changes in libido, can be perplexing to partners and family members who may not understand their cause. Discussing these changes openly can help your loved ones understand what you're going through and how they might support you.

Addressing Emotional and Psychological Changes

Menopause can also bring emotional and psychological changes. Women may experience mood swings, anxiety, or feelings of sadness. Sharing these experiences with family members and partners can help them understand the emotional challenges and offer appropriate support, whether it's providing space, a listening ear, or helping to find professional support if needed.

Communicating Needs and Boundaries

It's crucial to communicate your needs and boundaries clearly. This might involve explaining when you need some alone time, discussing changes in your sexual relationship, or expressing how best others can support you. Being clear about your needs can prevent misunderstandings and ensure that your support system is effective and responsive.

Educating Family Members about Menopause

Education plays a key role in effective communication. Sharing information about menopause with your partner and family can demystify the process and make it easier for them to understand and empathize with your experience. This could involve sharing articles, books, or even attending educational sessions together.

Navigating Changes in Sexual Relationships

Changes in sexual desire or response can be one of the more challenging aspects of menopause to discuss with a partner. It's important to approach these conversations with honesty and sensitivity. Discussing what feels good, what doesn't, and exploring new ways to maintain intimacy can be beneficial.

Managing Reactions and Misunderstandings

Reactions to these discussions can vary, and it's important to be prepared for a range of responses. Family members and partners might not always understand immediately. Patience and continuous dialogue can help in gradually building understanding and empathy.

Seeking Professional Guidance

In some cases, it might be helpful to seek guidance from a counselor or therapist, particularly if communication challenges are affecting the relationship. Couples counseling can provide a space for both partners to express their feelings and concerns with the guidance of a professional.

Supporting Each Other

Encouraging family members and partners to express their feelings and concerns about the changes they observe can foster mutual support. It's a two-way street where both sides need to feel heard and supported.

The Role of Emotional Support

Emotional support is a critical component of navigating menopause. Having a partner or family members who are understanding and empathetic can make a significant difference in how women experience and manage menopause.

Conclusion

Effective communication with partners and family members is crucial during the menopause transition. It involves not only sharing your experiences and needs but also educating and involving your loved ones in the process. Open and honest dialogue can foster understanding, empathy, and support, helping to maintain and even strengthen relationships during this significant life stage. By approaching these conversations with honesty, sensitivity, and a willingness to educate and listen, women can create a supportive environment that facilitates a more positive menopause experience.

Rekindling Intimacy and Maintaining Healthy Relationships

Menopause is often a period of significant change in a woman's life, and these changes can sometimes strain intimate and personal relationships. From physical symptoms like vaginal dryness and hot flashes to emotional challenges such as mood swings and decreased libido, menopause can impact the dynamics of relationships. However, with understanding, communication, and a few adjustments, it is possible to rekindle intimacy and maintain healthy relationships during this transition. This blog post will explore how to navigate these changes and strengthen relationships during menopause.

Understanding the Impact of Menopause on Relationships

Recognizing how menopause can affect relationships is the first step toward addressing its challenges. Hormonal changes can lead to decreased libido and discomfort during sex, while emotional fluctuations can create misunderstandings and communication barriers. Accepting that these changes are a normal part of menopause can help both partners develop a more empathetic and supportive approach.

Communication is Key

Open and honest communication is vital for maintaining a strong relationship during menopause. Discussing what you are going through, how it affects you, and your needs can help your partner understand your experience. This dialogue should also include discussing any changes in sexual desire or response, as well as exploring new ways to express intimacy and affection.

Redefining Intimacy

Intimacy is not limited to sexual activities; it encompasses a range of emotional and physical expressions. Menopause is an opportunity to explore different forms of intimacy, such as cuddling, massage, or simply spending quality time together. Finding new ways to connect that are mutually satisfying can strengthen your relationship.

Adjusting to Physical Changes

Physical changes during menopause, such as vaginal dryness, can make sexual activity uncomfortable. Using lubricants or vaginal moisturizers can help alleviate discomfort. In some cases, seeking medical advice for hormonal or non-hormonal treatments to address these issues can be beneficial.

Prioritizing Emotional Connection

Strengthening the emotional aspects of a relationship can bolster intimacy. Engaging in activities that foster closeness, sharing thoughts and feelings, and showing appreciation and affection can enhance the emotional bond between partners.

Dealing with Mood Swings

Mood swings and emotional changes can be challenging for both partners. Being patient, understanding, and supportive is important. It's also helpful to identify triggers and develop strategies to manage emotional fluctuations, such as practicing relaxation techniques or engaging in enjoyable activities.

Seeking Professional Help

If challenges in your relationship are becoming difficult to manage, seeking the help of a therapist or counselor can be a constructive step. Couples therapy can provide a safe space to explore issues and develop strategies to improve the relationship.

Maintaining Physical Health

A healthy lifestyle can positively impact sexual health and overall well-being. Regular exercise, a balanced diet, and adequate sleep can improve energy levels, body image, and mood, all of which contribute to a healthy relationship.

Fostering Independence

Maintaining individual interests and activities can be beneficial for both partners. Having separate hobbies and spending time apart can bring freshness and vitality to the relationship, enhancing the time spent together.

Exploring New Activities Together

Trying new activities or hobbies together can be a fun way to connect and deepen your relationship. Whether it's taking a class, traveling, or starting a new hobby, shared experiences can create new memories and strengthen bonds.

The Role of Patience and Understanding

Patience and understanding from both partners are crucial during menopause. Recognizing that adjustments take time and that empathy is key can help navigate the transition more smoothly.

Conclusion

Menopause can bring challenges to intimate and personal relationships, but with open communication, understanding, and a willingness to adapt, it is possible to maintain and even strengthen these bonds. Exploring new forms of intimacy, adjusting to physical changes, prioritizing emotional connection, and maintaining individuality are all important aspects of navigating relationships during menopause. By approaching this life stage with empathy, patience, and a willingness to grow together, couples can enjoy a fulfilling and supportive relationship through menopause and beyond.

Chapter 9: Planning for a Healthy Future

Preventative Health Measures Post-Menopause

Post-menopause marks a new chapter in a woman's life, accompanied by specific health concerns that require attention and care. The years following menopause can bring increased risks of certain health conditions, making preventative health measures more important than ever. This blog post will explore various preventative strategies that post-menopausal women can adopt to maintain their health and well-being.

Understanding the Health Risks Post-Menopause

After menopause, the decrease in estrogen levels can affect various aspects of health, leading to increased risks of osteoporosis, heart disease, and changes in weight and metabolism. Recognizing these risks is the first step in taking proactive measures to prevent potential health problems.

Osteoporosis and Bone Health

Osteoporosis, characterized by weakened bones, becomes a significant concern post-menopause. The decline in estrogen can lead to decreased bone density, increasing the risk of fractures. To combat this, a diet rich in calcium and vitamin D is essential. Foods high in calcium, such as dairy products, leafy green vegetables, and fortified foods, should be included in the diet. Vitamin D is also crucial for calcium absorption and bone health. While sunlight is a natural source of vitamin D, supplements may be necessary, especially in regions with limited sun exposure.

Incorporating weight-bearing exercises, such as walking, jogging, and strength training, can also help maintain bone density. These activities stimulate bone formation and strengthen muscles, supporting overall bone health.

Cardiovascular Health

The risk of heart disease increases post-menopause, partly due to the protective effects of estrogen on the heart and arteries diminishing. To maintain heart health, a balanced diet low in saturated fats and high in fruits, vegetables, whole grains, and lean proteins is recommended. Regular cardiovascular exercise, like brisk walking, swimming, or cycling, is also crucial. These activities help control weight, reduce blood pressure, and improve cholesterol levels.

Monitoring blood pressure and cholesterol levels regularly is important. High blood pressure and high cholesterol are risk factors for heart disease, so keeping these under control can significantly reduce the risk.

Managing Weight and Metabolism

Many women experience changes in weight and metabolism post-menopause. A slower metabolism can lead to weight gain, particularly around the abdomen. Managing weight through a healthy diet and regular exercise is key. Focusing on portion control, eating nutrient-dense foods, and avoiding excess sugar and processed foods can help maintain a healthy weight.

Regular Health Screenings

Regular health screenings become increasingly important post-menopause. These include mammograms for breast cancer screening, colonoscopies for colorectal cancer screening, and bone density tests for osteoporosis. Regular check-ups with a healthcare provider are also essential to monitor overall health and manage any emerging health issues.

Mental Health and Well-being

Mental health is just as important as physical health, especially during the post-menopausal years. The hormonal changes during menopause can affect mood and increase the risk of depression and anxiety. Staying socially active, pursuing hobbies and interests, and seeking professional help if experiencing symptoms of depression or anxiety are important for maintaining mental well-being.

Sleep Quality

Maintaining good sleep hygiene is crucial post-menopause. Many women experience sleep disturbances during and after menopause. To improve sleep quality, establishing a regular sleep schedule, creating a comfortable sleep environment, and avoiding stimulants like caffeine close to bedtime can be beneficial.

Lifestyle Choices

Lifestyle choices play a significant role in health post-menopause. Quitting smoking, if applicable, is one of the most important steps. Smoking increases the risk of many health problems, including heart disease, osteoporosis, and several types of cancer. Limiting alcohol intake is also advisable, as excessive alcohol consumption can impact bone health and increase the risk of various health issues.

Conclusion

Post-menopause is a time to focus on preventive health measures to maintain and enhance overall well-being. By understanding the specific health risks associated with this life stage and adopting strategies to mitigate these risks, women can enjoy a healthy and active post-menopausal life. Regular health screenings, a balanced diet, regular exercise, maintaining bone and heart health, and paying attention to mental and emotional well-being are all key components of a comprehensive approach to health after menopause. With the right care and attention, the post-menopausal years can be some of the most fulfilling and healthiest years of a woman's life.

Managing Other Age-Related Health Concerns

Menopause signifies not only the end of a woman's reproductive years but also a time when various age-related health concerns begin to emerge. It's a period where the body undergoes numerous changes, increasing the risk of certain health conditions. This blog post will explore how women can manage other age-related health concerns that often accompany menopause, focusing on a holistic approach to health and well-being.

Recognizing Age-Related Health Risks

As women age, especially during and after menopause, they face an increased risk of various health issues. These include osteoporosis, heart disease, diabetes, and certain types of cancer. Additionally, cognitive health can become a concern, along with issues like joint health and vision changes.

Cardiovascular Health

With aging and the decline in estrogen levels, women's risk of cardiovascular diseases increases. Maintaining a heart-healthy lifestyle is crucial. This involves eating a balanced diet rich in fruits, vegetables, whole grains, and lean proteins. Regular physical activity, such as brisk walking, swimming, or cycling, helps maintain a healthy weight and improves heart function. Monitoring blood pressure and cholesterol levels regularly and managing stress through relaxation techniques are also essential steps.

Bone Health and Osteoporosis Prevention

Bone density tends to decrease post-menopause, raising the risk of osteoporosis and fractures. To combat this, calcium and vitamin D intake should be a priority. Weight-bearing exercises like walking, jogging, and resistance training help strengthen bones. It's also important to get regular bone density screenings to monitor bone health and take preventive actions early.

Diabetes and Metabolism

Changes in metabolism and weight gain around the abdomen are common in menopausal women, which can increase the risk of type 2 diabetes. A diet low in sugar and refined carbs, regular exercise, and maintaining a healthy weight are key factors in managing this risk. Regular screenings for blood sugar levels can help in early detection and management of diabetes.

Cancer Awareness

The risk of certain cancers, such as breast, colon, and ovarian cancer, increases with age. Regular screenings, including mammograms, colonoscopies, and pelvic exams, are vital for early detection. Awareness of family history and discussing any genetic risks with a healthcare provider are also important.

Cognitive Health

Maintaining cognitive health is a growing concern for aging women. Engaging in mentally stimulating activities, maintaining social connections, and staying physically active can help preserve cognitive function. A diet rich in antioxidants and omega-3 fatty acids, found in foods like fish, nuts, and seeds, can also support brain health.

Joint Health and Mobility

Joint health can deteriorate with age, leading to conditions like osteoarthritis. Regular exercise, maintaining a healthy weight to reduce stress on joints, and incorporating anti-inflammatory foods into the diet can help maintain joint health and mobility.

Eye Health

Vision changes are common with aging, with risks of conditions like cataracts and glaucoma increasing. Regular eye exams are essential to detect any issues early. Protecting eyes from excessive sun exposure and ensuring a diet rich in vitamins A, C, and E can support eye health.

Skin Care

Aging affects skin health, leading to dryness, loss of elasticity, and wrinkles. A skincare routine that includes hydration, sun protection, and possibly the use of retinoids or other age-appropriate skin treatments can help maintain skin health. Staying hydrated and eating a diet rich in antioxidants can also support skin from the inside out.

Hearing Health

Hearing loss can also become a concern with age. Regular hearing check-ups can help in early detection and management. Protecting ears from prolonged loud noises and maintaining overall health can contribute to preserving hearing.

Mental and Emotional Well-being

Mental and emotional well-being is just as important as physical health. Menopause can be a time of significant emotional transition, and it's important to address any feelings of sadness, loss, or anxiety. Seeking support from friends, family, or professionals can help in navigating these emotional changes.

Holistic Approach to Health

Managing age-related health concerns post-menopause requires a holistic approach. This involves not only focusing on physical health but also paying attention to mental, emotional, and social well-being. Regular check-ups, a healthy lifestyle, and being proactive about screenings and preventive care are key components of managing health during this stage of life.

Conclusion

Navigating the post-menopausal years and managing age-related health concerns requires awareness, proactive care, and a holistic approach to health. By understanding the increased risks and taking steps to address them, women can maintain their health and enjoy a vibrant, active life post-menopause. Regular health screenings, a balanced diet, regular exercise, and attention to mental and emotional well-being are all crucial in managing the various aspects of health during this important stage of life.

Embracing Aging Positively and Healthily

Menopause marks a significant milestone in the aging process, one that often brings mixed emotions. While it can be a challenging time due to the various physical and emotional changes it entails, menopause also presents an opportunity to embrace aging positively and healthily. This blog post aims to explore how women can approach aging with a positive mindset and healthy practices, turning menopause into a period of growth, self-discovery, and well-being.

Understanding the Aging Process

Aging is a natural part of life, and menopause is one of its key stages for women. It's important to understand that aging is not just about physical changes; it also encompasses wisdom, experiences, and growth. By accepting aging as a natural and inevitable process, women can approach menopause with a more positive and proactive mindset.

Shifting Perspectives on Aging

Challenging the societal stereotypes and personal beliefs about aging can help women view this phase of life more positively. Aging is often associated with loss, but it can also be a time of gaining–gaining more time for oneself, new hobbies, and different experiences. Focusing on the positives that come with age, such as wisdom, confidence, and a better understanding of oneself, can shift the perspective from fear and negativity to optimism and acceptance.

Prioritizing Health and Wellness

Taking care of physical health is crucial as women age. This means adopting a balanced diet, engaging in regular physical activity, getting adequate sleep, and keeping up with regular health

screenings. A healthy lifestyle not only helps in managing menopause symptoms but also reduces the risk of age-related diseases
and improves overall quality of life.

Embracing Mental and Emotional Health

Mental and emotional health is just as important as physical health
during menopause. Practices such as mindfulness, meditation,
and yoga can help manage stress and promote mental well-being.
Seeking social support, whether through friends, family, or support
groups, can also provide emotional comfort and a sense of community.

Lifelong Learning and Growth

Menopause can be a great time to pursue interests and activities
that there may not have been time for earlier in life. Engaging in
lifelong learning, whether it's taking up a new hobby, enrolling in
courses, or traveling, can provide intellectual stimulation and joy.

Focusing on Relationships

This stage of life can also be an opportunity to nurture relationships with family and friends or build new ones. Strengthening
these social ties can provide emotional support, enhance happiness, and contribute to a sense of belonging and purpose.

Exploring New Opportunities

Menopause often coincides with other life changes, such as
children leaving home or retirement. This can be an opportunity
to explore new roles, reinvent oneself, or engage in new activities
that bring fulfillment and joy.

Cultivating a Positive Body Image

Changes in body shape and appearance are common during
menopause. Cultivating a positive body image by focusing on the
body's strengths and abilities, rather than its perceived flaws, can
promote self-esteem and body positivity.

Keeping a Sense of Humor

Maintaining a sense of humor and being able to laugh at oneself can be a powerful tool in dealing with the challenges of aging. Humor can lighten difficult situations and help maintain a positive outlook on life.

Giving Back and Volunteering

Volunteering or giving back to the community can be a rewarding way to spend time during and after menopause. It can provide a sense of purpose, help build connections, and have a positive impact on mental and emotional health.

Self-Reflection and Acceptance

Menopause is a good time for self-reflection and acceptance. Embracing the changes that come with aging, acknowledging accomplishments, and being kind to oneself can lead to a more fulfilling and content life stage.

Conclusion

Embracing aging positively and healthily during and after menopause is about more than just dealing with physical changes; it's about a holistic approach to life. By focusing on physical, mental, and emotional health, engaging in lifelong learning, nurturing relationships, and maintaining a positive outlook, women can transform their menopause years into a period of growth, happiness, and well-being. This life stage can be an opportunity to celebrate the journey so far and look forward to the experiences and wisdom that come with age.

Chapter 10: Stories from the Journey

Personal Stories and Experiences from Diverse Women

Menopause is a universal experience for women, yet each woman's journey through this significant life transition is unique. This blog post aims to share personal stories and experiences from diverse women, highlighting the myriad ways menopause can be experienced and navigated. These stories reflect the varied emotional, physical, and psychological landscapes of menopause, offering insights and perspectives that can enrich our understanding of this complex phase of life.

Embracing Change: Maria's Story

Maria, a 52-year-old teacher from Mexico, began experiencing menopausal symptoms in her late 40s. Initially, she struggled with hot flashes and sleep disturbances, which made her daily routine challenging. However, Maria found solace in her close-knit family and cultural traditions that celebrated aging as a natural and respected part of life. She embraced herbal remedies passed down through generations, which helped alleviate some of her symptoms. For Maria, menopause became an opportunity to reconnect with her heritage and discover the wisdom that comes with age.

Finding Balance: Aisha's Journey

Aisha, a 48-year-old software engineer from Nigeria, encountered menopause earlier than she expected. The onset of symptoms coincided with a demanding period in her career, creating a stressful combination. Aisha turned to yoga and meditation, practices she had never considered before, to manage her stress and mood swings. These mind-body practices not only helped her navigate menopause more smoothly but also brought a newfound sense of balance and calm to her life, impacting her both personally and professionally.

Challenging Stereotypes: Li's Experience

Li, a 55-year-old business owner from China, faced menopause with determination to challenge the stereotypes and stigma around aging in women. She openly discussed her menopause experience with friends and colleagues, breaking the cultural taboo surrounding the topic. Li's willingness to share her story encouraged other women in her community to speak out and seek support, fostering a more open dialogue about women's health and aging.

Rediscovering Self: Emma's Transformation

Emma, a 50-year-old artist from the United States, found menopause to be a period of profound self-discovery. The transition pushed her to reevaluate her life, leading to significant changes in her personal and professional world. Emma used art to express and process her feelings, finding that her work gained depth and emotion as she navigated the ups and downs of menopause. For her, menopause was a catalyst for rediscovering her passion and creativity.

Seeking Support: Fatima's Approach

Fatima, a 53-year-old community leader from Pakistan, experienced severe mood swings and depression during menopause. Recognizing the need for support, she sought help from a women's health counselor, a decision that was initially met with skepticism in her community. However, Fatima's positive experience with counseling changed not only her approach to menopause but also influenced other women in her community to seek professional help for their health concerns.

Embracing New Chapters: Susan's Adventure

Susan, a 57-year-old retiree from Australia, saw menopause as the beginning of a new adventure. With her children grown and a newfound freedom in retirement, she embarked on travels and hobbies she had previously set aside. Susan's story is a testament to the opportunities that menopause can present, turning a potentially challenging time into a period of exploration and joy.

Cultural Wisdom: Sunita's Lessons

Sunita, a 60-year-old teacher from India, leaned on the wisdom of Ayurveda to manage her menopause symptoms. She adopted a diet and lifestyle in line with her Ayurvedic constitution, which helped alleviate her hot flashes and insomnia. Sunita's experience highlights the importance of cultural practices and traditional wisdom in managing menopause.

Conclusion

These personal stories from diverse women around the world showcase the myriad ways in which menopause can be experienced and managed. They reflect resilience, transformation, cultural wisdom, and the pursuit of balance and well-being. Each story contributes to a richer understanding of menopause, reminding us that while it is a universal experience, it is also deeply personal and individual. Sharing and listening to these experiences can provide comfort, inspiration, and a sense of community for women navigating this significant life transition.

Tips and Advice from Those Who've Navigated Menopause Successfully

Menopause, a natural part of aging, can be a challenging time for many women. However, with the right approach and mindset, it's possible to navigate this transition successfully and even find new joys in this stage of life. This blog post gathers tips and advice from women who have navigated menopause successfully, offering practical and empowering insights for those currently going through this journey.

Embrace the Change

One of the key pieces of advice from women who have successfully navigated menopause is to embrace the change rather than resist it. Accepting menopause as a natural and inevitable part of life can help in approaching it with a positive mindset. Seeing it as a time for growth and new opportunities rather than just a series of symptoms to be endured can make a significant difference.

Stay Informed and Be Proactive

Staying informed about what to expect during menopause is crucial. Understanding the potential physical and emotional changes can prepare you for what's ahead. Being proactive about your health during this time is also important. Regular health check-ups, being aware of the risk of conditions like osteoporosis and heart disease, and taking preventative steps are vital.

Cultivate a Supportive Network

Having a supportive network of friends, family, or others going through similar experiences is invaluable. Sharing your experiences, concerns, and tips with others can provide comfort, practical advice, and a sense of community. Some women find joining support groups or online forums particularly helpful.

Prioritize Self-Care

Self-care becomes even more important during menopause. This includes eating a balanced diet, staying active, getting enough sleep, and managing stress. Many women find that activities like yoga, meditation, or simply spending time in nature can significantly improve their mood and overall well-being.

Open Communication with Partners

Open communication with your partner is essential, especially regarding how menopause is affecting your relationship, including your sex life. Discussing changes in your body, sexual needs, and emotional state can help maintain intimacy and understanding in your relationship.

Explore New Interests and Hobbies

Menopause can be a great time to explore new interests or revisit old hobbies. Engaging in activities that bring joy and fulfillment can be a great way to navigate through this transition. Whether it's painting, writing, traveling, or any other pursuit, finding something that you love doing can be immensely rewarding.

Seek Professional Help When Needed

Don't hesitate to seek professional help if you're struggling with menopause symptoms. This can include talking to a doctor about hormone replacement therapy (HRT) or other treatments, seeing a therapist to address emotional challenges, or consulting a dietitian for nutritional advice.

Stay Physically Active

Regular exercise is not only good for physical health but also for emotional and mental well-being. It can help manage symptoms like hot flashes, improve sleep, and reduce the risk of anxiety and depression. Activities like walking, swimming, or cycling can be particularly beneficial.

Focus on the Positive

Focusing on the positive aspects of menopause, like no longer having periods or not having to worry about pregnancy, can help maintain a positive outlook. Many women also find that they gain a greater sense of confidence and self-awareness during this time.

Practice Mindfulness and Meditation

Mindfulness and meditation can help manage stress and improve emotional well-being. Practices that encourage living in the moment and finding peace within oneself can be particularly helpful during the menopause transition.

Keep a Sense of Humor

Having a sense of humor and being able to laugh at the challenges can be a great coping mechanism. Humor can lighten the mood and make it easier to deal with difficult situations.

Embrace Your Age and Experience

Recognize the wisdom, experience, and strength that come with age. Many women find that they feel more confident and assured in their post-menopausal years. Embracing your age and all that comes with it can be empowering.

Conclusion

Navigating menopause successfully often means embracing change, staying informed, prioritizing self-care, maintaining a supportive network, and focusing on the positive. Each woman's experience with menopause is unique, but these tips and advice from those who've been through it can provide guidance and reassurance. Approaching menopause as a natural part of life's journey, with its own challenges and rewards, can lead to a more fulfilling and joyful experience.

Chapter 11: Resources and Tools for the Journey

Checklists and Charts for Tracking Symptoms and Health

Navigating menopause can often feel like trying to find your way through a maze without a map. However, creating checklists and charts to track symptoms and health can be an effective way to gain insights into your menopausal journey. Such tools not only help in understanding your body's changes but also provide valuable information for discussions with healthcare providers. In this blog post, we will discuss how to create and utilize checklists and charts to effectively monitor menopause symptoms and overall health.

The Importance of Tracking Menopause Symptoms

Menopause brings a variety of symptoms that can fluctuate in intensity and frequency. Tracking these symptoms can help identify patterns, triggers, and what alleviates them. This information is crucial not only for self-awareness but also for informing healthcare decisions.

Creating a Symptom Checklist

A symptom checklist for menopause should include common symptoms like hot flashes, night sweats, sleep disturbances, mood swings, and changes in menstrual patterns. It can also include other symptoms such as weight changes, joint pain, headaches, and changes in libido. Each day, you can check off the symptoms you experience and note their severity. This can provide a clear picture over time of how menopause is affecting you.

Using a Symptom Chart for Detailed Tracking

For a more detailed analysis, a symptom chart can be helpful. This chart can include columns for each day of the month and rows for different symptoms. You can rate the severity of each symptom on a scale (such as 1-5) each day. This method allows you to visually track the frequency and intensity of your symptoms over time.

Monitoring Menstrual Patterns

During the perimenopausal phase, menstrual patterns can change significantly. Keeping track of your menstrual cycle, including the length, flow, and any irregularities, can be important. This information can help in identifying the transition into menopause and can be valuable during medical consultations.

Charting Lifestyle Factors

Lifestyle factors such as diet, exercise, stress levels, and sleep patterns can greatly influence menopause symptoms. Including these in your charts or checklists can help identify what lifestyle changes might improve your symptoms. For instance, you might notice that certain foods trigger hot flashes or that exercise improves your mood.

Tracking Emotional and Mental Health

Menopause can also affect your emotional and mental well-being. Tracking your emotional state can help you understand if your symptoms are having an impact on your mental health. This can include noting feelings of anxiety, depression, irritability, or changes in mood.

Utilizing Health Apps

There are several health apps available that can simplify tracking menopause symptoms. These apps can provide templates for checklists and charts, making it easier to record and analyze your symptoms. Some apps also offer additional features like reminders to take medications or attend medical appointments.

Keeping a Health Journal

In addition to checklists and charts, keeping a health journal can be beneficial. In this journal, you can write more detailed entries about your day-to-day experiences with menopause, including how you're feeling emotionally and physically. This can provide deeper insights into your overall well-being.

Sharing Information with Healthcare Providers

The information gathered from your checklists, charts, and journal can be extremely helpful during appointments with your healthcare providers. It can help your doctor understand your experience of menopause more accurately and tailor their advice and treatment to your specific needs.

Reviewing and Adjusting Over Time

As menopause is a transition over several years, your symptoms and health needs may change over time. Regularly reviewing your checklists and charts can help you adjust your strategies for managing menopause. It can also be encouraging to see improvements or positive changes as a result of lifestyle adjustments or treatments.

Conclusion

Creating and utilizing checklists and charts to track menopause symptoms and health can empower you to understand and manage this phase of life more effectively. By documenting your experiences, you gain valuable insights into your body's changes, which can inform your healthcare decisions and help you advocate for your health needs. This approach not only enhances self-awareness but also fosters a proactive attitude toward managing menopause.

Directory of Resources: Websites, Support Groups, Books

Navigating menopause can be made easier with access to the right resources. From informative websites and supportive community groups to insightful books, there are numerous avenues available for women seeking guidance, information, or simply a sense of community during this transition. This blog post aims to provide a directory of resources for those experiencing menopause, offering a range of options to suit different needs and preferences.

Informative Websites

The internet offers a wealth of information on menopause, providing details on symptoms, treatments, and lifestyle tips.

- **Women's Health Websites**: Many health websites have dedicated sections for menopause, offering articles, tips, and expert advice. These sites are often run by healthcare professionals and provide medically accurate information.

- **Menopause-Specific Portals**: There are websites specifically focused on menopause, offering comprehensive information covering all aspects of this life stage. These platforms often include FAQs, expert interviews, and the latest research updates.

- **Health Forums and Blogs**: Online forums and blogs can be a rich source of personal stories and experiences. While they offer more subjective insights, they can be comforting and provide a sense of community.

Support Groups

Support groups, whether online or in-person, provide a platform for women to share their experiences and advice.

- **Local Community Groups**: Many communities have support groups for women going through menopause. These groups often meet regularly, providing a space to share experiences and tips in a supportive environment.

- **Online Forums and Social Media**: Online support groups and forums offer the convenience of connecting with others from the comfort of your home. Social media platforms like Facebook or Reddit have specific groups or communities dedicated to menopause support.

Recommended Books

A range of books on menopause can offer insights, advice, and comfort. These books often cover medical advice, personal stories, and lifestyle tips.

- **Medical and Holistic Health Books**: Authored by healthcare professionals, these books provide detailed information on the medical aspects of menopause, including symptom management and treatment options.

- **Personal Narratives and Memoirs**: Books written by women who have gone through menopause can offer personal insights and relatable experiences. These narratives often combine humor, advice, and comfort.

- **Lifestyle and Wellness Guides**: Focusing on diet, exercise, and mental well-being, these guides offer practical tips for managing menopause symptoms and maintaining overall health.

Educational Videos and Podcasts

Videos and podcasts are increasingly popular formats for information and support.

- **Medical Expert Videos and Webinars**: Many health websites and platforms host educational videos and webinars led by medical experts. These can be a great way to stay informed about the latest research and advice.

- **Podcasts on Women's Health**: There are podcasts dedicated to menopause and women's health, featuring expert interviews, Q&A sessions, and discussions on various menopause-related topics.

Health and Wellness Apps

Several apps are designed to help women navigate menopause, offering symptom tracking, lifestyle tips, and more.

- **Symptom Trackers and Health Apps**: These apps allow women to track their menopause symptoms, monitor their health, and sometimes connect with a community or health professionals.
- **Meditation and Mindfulness Apps**: Apps focusing on meditation and mindfulness can be particularly useful for managing stress, sleep issues, and mood swings associated with menopause.

Professional Organizations and Associations

Professional organizations dedicated to menopause and women's health can be valuable resources for information and support.

- **National and International Menopause Societies**: These organizations offer resources, research updates, and sometimes directories of healthcare providers specializing in menopause.
- **Women's Health Advocacy Groups**: These groups focus on broader aspects of women's health, including menopause, and often engage in advocacy and awareness initiatives.

Conclusion

The journey through menopause is unique for each woman, but having access to a diverse range of resources can make it more manageable and less isolating. Whether it's through informative websites, supportive groups, insightful books, podcasts, or health apps, there are numerous tools available to help women navigate this life stage. These resources offer not only valuable information and tips but also a sense of community and understanding, reminding women that they are not alone in their menopause experience.

Final Thoughts: Empowerment Through Knowledge and Community

Menopause, a natural part of every woman's life journey, often comes with its own set of challenges and changes. However, it also presents an opportunity for empowerment through knowledge and community. As we conclude this series on navigating menopause, it's crucial to reflect on how understanding and support can transform this life stage into a period of growth and empowerment. This final blog post aims to encapsulate the essence of finding strength, resilience, and camaraderie during menopause.

Embracing Menopause with Knowledge

Knowledge is a powerful tool in managing menopause effectively. Understanding the physiological changes that occur during this time helps demystify the process and prepares women to deal with symptoms and changes more confidently. It's important to stay informed about various aspects of menopause, from symptom management to long-term health considerations. This knowledge not only empowers women to make informed decisions about their health but also helps in addressing any fears or misconceptions.

Educational resources such as books, medical websites, and seminars provide valuable information. Being aware of the latest research and treatment options allows women to engage in more meaningful discussions with their healthcare providers, ensuring they receive care that aligns with their individual needs and preferences.

The Power of Community

The role of community in navigating menopause cannot be overstated. Sharing experiences with others who are going through similar changes fosters a sense of solidarity and understanding. Support groups, whether online or in person, offer spaces where women can express their feelings, share advice, and find comfort in the shared experience of menopause.

These communities can also be a source of diverse perspectives, offering insights into how women from different backgrounds and cultures experience and manage menopause. Learning from these diverse experiences can broaden understanding and provide a range of strategies for coping with menopause.

Building a Supportive Network

Creating a network of support with friends, family, and healthcare providers is essential. Open communication with loved ones about the challenges and changes experienced during menopause can help in building a supportive environment at home. Healthcare providers, including gynecologists, therapists, and nutritionists, play a crucial role in providing professional guidance and support.

Empowerment Through Self-Care

Empowerment during menopause also comes from prioritizing self-care. This includes not only taking care of physical health through diet and exercise but also paying attention to emotional and mental well-being. Practices like yoga, meditation, and mindfulness can help manage stress and foster a sense of inner peace. Pursuing hobbies, engaging in activities that bring joy, and taking time for relaxation are also vital aspects of self-care.

Advocacy and Raising Awareness

Becoming an advocate for menopause awareness is another form of empowerment. By sharing personal experiences, raising awareness about menopause-related issues, and advocating for better healthcare and support, women can help break the stigma and silence that often surrounds this topic. This advocacy can also drive better research, resources, and policies related to women's health.

The Importance of Lifelong Learning

Menopause is also a time for continued learning and personal development. Exploring new interests, learning new skills, or engaging in educational pursuits can keep the mind active and contribute to a fulfilling life. Lifelong learning can be both a form of self-care and a way to stay engaged and stimulated during and after the menopausal transition.

Embracing Change and New Beginnings

Finally, menopause can be viewed as a period of change and new beginnings. It's a time when women can reassess their lives, goals, and what brings them happiness. Embracing this phase as an opportunity for growth and new experiences can lead to a more positive and enriching menopause journey.

Conclusion

Menopause, with all its challenges, also brings opportunities for empowerment, growth, and connection. Through gaining knowledge, building a supportive community, prioritizing self-care, and embracing new beginnings, women can navigate this transition with strength and confidence. Empowerment through menopause is about understanding, accepting, and making the most of this life stage, turning it into a period of positive transformation and fulfillment.

Chapter 12: Conclusion

Reflecting on Menopause as a Transition, Not an Ending

Menopause, often framed in the context of an ending — the end of fertility and the close of a certain chapter of womanhood — is, in many ways, more accurately characterized as a transition. It's a significant shift, yes, but also a passage into a new phase of life rich with its own unique possibilities and experiences. This blog post aims to reframe menopause not as an ending, but as a transition, offering a perspective that celebrates the growth, wisdom, and new opportunities it brings.

Menopause: A New Beginning

The cessation of menstruation and the reproductive years can often be viewed with a sense of loss. However, this period also marks the beginning of something new. Post-menopause, many women report a newfound sense of freedom, liberation from the monthly cycles, and a renewed focus on self-care and personal growth. This time can be an invitation to explore new interests, deepen self-awareness, and engage in life from a more centered and experienced perspective.

Reassessing and Realigning Life Goals

Menopause often coincides with other life changes, such as children growing up and moving out or reaching milestones in careers. This juncture provides an opportunity to reassess life goals and aspirations. For many women, this period becomes a time to realign their paths and pursue passions or interests that might have been on hold.

Embracing Wisdom and Experience

With age comes wisdom and a wealth of life experience. Menopause can be a time to embrace this wisdom, using it to guide decisions, foster relationships, and impart knowledge to younger generations. It's a stage where the insights gained from years of experience come to fruition, offering a deeper understanding of life and oneself.

Navigating Physical Changes with Grace

While menopause brings physical changes that can be challenging, it also offers an opportunity to approach these changes with grace and acceptance. It's a time to honor the body for all it has been through and continues to go through. Adopting a healthy lifestyle, focusing on nutrition, exercise, and mental well-being, can transform this period into one of rejuvenation and vitality.

A Time for Renewed Relationships

Menopause can also be a time to renew and deepen relationships. With a different perspective on life, relationships with partners, family, and friends can evolve in more meaningful ways. It also presents an opportunity to form new connections, especially with those who share similar experiences and understand the nuances of this life stage.

The Power of Community and Shared Experiences

Finding community during menopause can be incredibly empowering. Sharing experiences with others who are at the same stage can provide support, understanding, and a sense of belonging. It's comforting and affirming to know that one is not alone in this journey.

Self-Discovery and Personal Development

This transition can spark a journey of self-discovery and personal development. Many women use this time to explore aspects of themselves that they may have neglected or not had the opportunity to focus on before. This can include spiritual pursuits, creative endeavors, or educational interests.

Menopause as a Cultural Shift

Menopause is also prompting a cultural shift, challenging the societal norms and stereotypes around aging and women's health. By openly discussing and embracing menopause, there's an opportunity to change the narrative, creating a more positive and empowering dialogue around this natural life stage.

The Importance of Mental and Emotional Health

Recognizing and nurturing mental and emotional health is crucial during menopause. This period can bring a range of emotions, from grief and loss to relief and excitement. Attending to mental health through practices like mindfulness, counseling, or simply engaging in enjoyable activities can be key to a positive transition.

Looking Forward with Optimism

Approaching menopause with optimism and a forward-looking attitude can set the tone for this new phase of life. It's a chance to model resilience and positivity, showing that life post-menopause can be fulfilling, vibrant, and rich with opportunities.

Conclusion

Menopause, rather than being an ending, is a transition to a new phase of life filled with potential. It offers opportunities for growth, self-discovery, and deepening connections with others. By embracing this transition with positivity, resilience, and an open mind, women can experience menopause as a meaningful and empowering journey, one that opens the door to new beginnings and experiences.

The Ongoing Journey: Life After Menopause

Menopause, often viewed as a significant milestone, is not just an end to the reproductive years but also the beginning of a new and potentially enriching phase of life. The post-menopausal period can be a time of great personal growth, new opportunities, and deepened self-awareness. This blog post aims to shed light on the ongoing journey of life after menopause, highlighting the opportunities, changes, and experiences that characterize this stage.

Embracing a New Phase of Life

The post-menopausal years offer a chance to embrace a new phase of life with enthusiasm and positivity. Freed from the cyclical nature of menstruation, many women find a new sense of liberation and opportunity. This period can be seen as a blank canvas, ready to be filled with new experiences, adventures, and personal growth.

Health and Wellness in Focus

Post-menopause brings about a shift in health priorities. With an increased risk of conditions such as osteoporosis and heart disease, focusing on health and wellness becomes even more important. This includes maintaining a balanced diet, regular exercise, and regular health screenings. It's also a time to focus on mental health, recognizing the importance of emotional well-being and the role it plays in overall health.

Pursuing Passions and Interests

For many women, the post-menopausal years can be a time to pursue passions and interests that may have been put on hold. Whether it's travel, starting a new business, diving into a creative hobby, or going back to school, this period offers the freedom and time to explore these pursuits fully.

Deepening Relationships and Building New Ones

Life after menopause can also be a time for deepening existing relationships and building new ones. With a more mature perspective on life, relationships with partners, friends, and family can take on new depths. It's also a great time to meet new people, form new friendships, and expand social circles.

The Wisdom of Experience

One of the greatest gifts of this stage of life is the wisdom that comes from years of experience. Many women find they are more confident, self-assured, and in tune with their needs and desires. This wisdom can be shared with younger generations, providing guidance and support, or it can be used to navigate the new challenges and opportunities that arise.

Exploring New Forms of Creativity and Expression

Post-menopause can be a highly creative time. With life experience as a backdrop, many women find new ways to express themselves, whether through writing, art, music, or other creative endeavors. This creativity can be a source of joy, fulfillment, and a powerful way to tell one's own story.

Engaging in Community and Volunteer Work

Many post-menopausal women find fulfillment in engaging with their communities or in volunteer work. This engagement can provide a sense of purpose, connection, and the satisfaction of giving back. It can also be a way to utilize professional skills in a new, rewarding context.

Staying Curious and Open to Learning

The post-menopausal years can be a time of continued learning and curiosity. This might mean taking up new hobbies, traveling to new places, or simply staying open to new ideas and experiences. Lifelong learning can keep the mind active and engaged, contributing to a richer, more fulfilling life.

Prioritizing Self-Care and Personal Growth

Self-care takes on a new importance post-menopause. This includes not only physical care but also taking the time for personal growth, reflection, and self-discovery. It's a time to listen to one's own needs and to prioritize activities that bring personal joy and satisfaction.

Reflecting and Planning for the Future

Post-menopause is also a time to reflect on past achievements and to plan for the future. This might involve considering retirement plans, lifestyle changes, or setting new goals and aspirations. It's a period to look back with pride and forward with anticipation.

Conclusion

Life after menopause is an ongoing journey, filled with opportunities for growth, discovery, and fulfillment. By embracing this stage with a positive and proactive approach, focusing on health and well-being, pursuing passions, deepening relationships, and staying open to new experiences, women can enjoy a vibrant and enriching post-menopausal life. This period is not just an ending but a continuation of the journey, offering its own unique rewards and experiences.